Simply Local Flaps

W0050405

Michael F. Klaassen · Earle Brown
Felix Behan

Simply Local Flaps

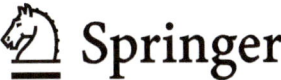

Michael F. Klaassen
New Face Surgery Clinic
Epsom, Auckland
New Zealand

Felix Behan
Former Head of Plastic Surgery Unit,
Western Hospital
Former Principal Reconstructive Surgeon
in Head and Neck Service
Peter MacCallum Cancer Centre
Melbourne, Victoria
Australia

Earle Brown
Former Head of Plastic Surgery Unit
and former Clinical Director of Surgery
Middlemore Hospital
Auckland
New Zealand

The books from 2011 and 2016 were self-published by the authors.
ISBN 978-3-030-09643-4   ISBN 978-3-319-59400-2   (eBook)
https://doi.org/10.1007/978-3-319-59400-2

© Springer International Publishing AG 2018
Softcover re-print of the Hardcover 1st edition 2018
This work is subject to copyright. All rights are reserved by the Publisher, whether the whole or part of
the material is concerned, specifically the rights of translation, reprinting, reuse of illustrations, recita-
tion, broadcasting, reproduction on microfilms or in any other physical way, and transmission or information storage and retrieval, electronic adaptation, computer software, or by similar or dissimilar
methodology now known or hereafter developed.
The use of general descriptive names, registered names, trademarks, service marks, etc. in this publication does not imply, even in the absence of a specific statement, that such names are exempt from the
relevant protective laws and regulations and therefore free for general use.
The publisher, the authors and the editors are safe to assume that the advice and information in this book
are believed to be true and accurate at the date of publication. Neither the publisher nor the authors or the
editors give a warranty, express or implied, with respect to the material contained herein or for any errors
or omissions that may have been made. The publisher remains neutral with regard to jurisdictional claims
in published maps and institutional affiliations.

Printed on acid-free paper

This Springer imprint is published by Springer Nature
The registered company is Springer International Publishing AG
The registered company address is: Gewerbestrasse 11, 6330 Cham, Switzerland

Foreword

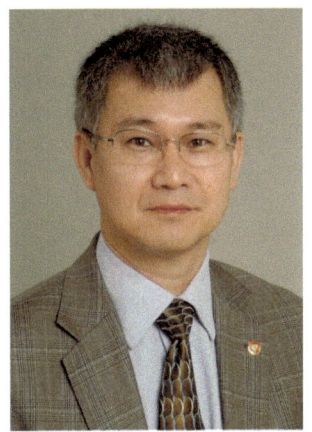

Dr. Swee T. Tan

Dr. Michael Klaassen, FRACS, encouraged, egged on and supported by close colleagues and co-authors Drs. Earle Brown and Felix Behan, has produced *Simply Local Flaps*. It is a privilege and a pleasure for me to be one of the first to view their work and to pen a foreword for this wonderful publication. The book consists of an extensive catalogue of pre-, intra- and post-operative photos of patients who have benefitted from local flap surgery that has preserved and/or restored their quality of life. This masterpiece, preceded by their previous publications, *Introduction to Local Flaps: A Surgeon's Handbook* and *Defining Local Flaps: Clinical Applications and Methods*, underscores how one thinks like a plastic surgeon when faced with varied and often challenging clinical scenarios. It will be a timeless treasure in the collection of both students and experienced practitioners of plastic surgery.

The 200 pages cover 125 clinical cases, mostly pertaining to the reconstruction of cutaneous defects following excision of skin cancers. This atlas is a practical guide that covers almost all possible situations faced by a busy practising plastic surgeon, drawn from a wealth of personal experience over many years of caring for patients. Yet it is not designed as a recipe-like cookbook. Underlying these apparent 'simple' cases and the challenging situations are the real gems, words of wisdom, nuances and the espousal of the fundamental surgical principles that underscore the elegant execution of operations characterised by a creative and innovative flair.

In addition, readers are treated to beautiful drawings and many diagrams, including those in the first part that help convey flap design and planning underpinned by fundamental guiding principles and sound decision-making. Many of these principles have been passed on from the greats and the wise, such as Gillies and McIndoe, through successive generations of plastic surgeons.

Execution of the operative plans has been illustrated in a coherent, stepwise and concise manner. The book highlights the hallmarks of a mature surgeon embarking on this area of surgical endeavour, characterised by a deep understanding of the difference between surgical principles and surgical technique. This book contains a roadmap and a toolbox, intricately and seamlessly linked but distinctive.

The early chapters of this book provide a useful framework for categorising local flaps by their composition, blood supply, geometry and means of transfer. As closure of the donor site and the resultant scars are critical aspects of a good design, the concepts behind identification of relaxed skin tension lines are emphasised, the clear objective being to achieve the best long-term results for the patient.

The book is divided into four parts interposed by beautiful artwork.

The three chapters in Part I are dedicated to the fundamentals—the basics, how to get started and technical tips. It also includes advice relating to wound care and scar management. These practical pointers are very useful to the novice and a reminder to the experienced practitioners, emphasising the importance of creating an environment of safe practice and good habits.

Part II consists of eight chapters describing the types of flaps that are traditionally taught and the ten most common flaps. These are tried and tested and time honoured, not just in relation to the size but also in dealing with challenging and complex defects. It contains various modifications of the original design and combinations of concepts that can be applied to unique situations. Chap. 9 in this part also includes a practical guide to W-plasty, Z-plasty and various modifications that can be applied not only to scar revision but also for the closure of the donor sites. Chap. 11 presents the most recommended ten traditional local flaps regarded by the authors, applied mostly to defects on the head and neck area.

The first two chapters of Part III are devoted to the keystone perforator island flap, first described and popularised by Dr. Felix Behan with application of this flap to various body sites, offering elegant solutions to some tricky situations. The second chapter of this part illustrates the application of keystone flaps to ten different parts of the body with clinical cases, as favoured by the lead author. The last chapter is dedicated to various combinations of flaps applied to many different and often very challenging situations.

The four chapters in Part IV are focused on judgement, decision-making and experience: essentially how to decide if a skin graft is better, matters relating to aesthetics, dealing with complications and how to think like a plastic surgeon. Chap. 17, which deals with surgical complications and their management, would arguably have been the most challenging chapter to write. Yet much can be learnt about pitfalls and how best to minimise the risk of complications and about management of them with courage and humility, particularly in supporting the patients through what can be a very difficult time.

Behind the beautiful outcome of the procedures, elegantly expressed on paper, lies the complex decision-making process that is second nature to good surgeons, in turn reflecting the judgement and wisdom accumulated over many years (being over 100 years collectively between the three eminent surgical practitioners).

The integrating theme of this book is about closing cutaneous defects with like tissues by using the adjacent area(s) of spare tissue and choosing the most efficient way of transfer whilst simultaneously achieving primary closure of the donor site (in most circumstances). There are occasions where other techniques such as skin grafting may offer an overall satisfactory and/or preferred solution. Underlying the application of all the techniques are sound principles that allow the display of creativity and innovation of plastic surgery, which is inherently a problem-solving specialty. In this way, and with imagination, the practitioner of the art of plastic surgery is equipped to design an operation that is suitable for every situation and every day.

Finally, the number of patients who have consented to their photographs being included in the book is a fitting testimony of their gratitude to the treating surgeon. The excellent outcome is the result of having a deeply grounded understanding of the principles, allowing appropriate surgical techniques to be applied to a particular clinical context. I am honoured by the invitation to express my views on this masterpiece. I have no doubt that other readers will also greatly enjoy and be enlightened by this outstanding contribution to the exciting and vital field of plastic surgery.

Swee T. Tan, ONZM, MBBS, PhD, FRACS
Gillies McIndoe Research Institute
Wellington, New Zealand

Preface

The background to this book is plastic surgery training and education. Dr. Earle Brown, FRACS, has been influencing me in this vein for 36 years and continues to do so. The principle of repairing like with like is one of the first lessons that the plastic surgery trainee learns. This principle is nowhere better illustrated than in the surgical practice of local flap repair. In the 1970s, a formal plastic surgery training programme was established at Middlemore Hospital in Auckland. Dr. Brown gathered a large collection of copied journal and textbook articles on local flap repairs. An attempt was made to sort them into a logical classification. The script of the original manual was typed on a typewriter, and the diagrams were cut from the copied articles and pasted in the gaps of the script—a forerunner of the computer term 'cut and paste'. These notes were photocopied and eventually issued to all new plastic surgery registrars.

I benefitted from these notes in 1986, when I commenced my formal plastic surgery training at Middlemore Hospital. Earle kept the original manual and gave me the faded typed pages contained in a large, weathered brown paper envelope in 2010. We collaborated as authors and in 2011 with the help of others produced *Introduction to Local Flaps: A Surgeon's Handbook.* Five years on and Earle suggested a sequel. We had omitted to acknowledge the keystone flap of our Australian friend, Associate Professor Felix Behan. Instead of a second edition, I had in mind to write something of a flap book atlas. This would include lots of images to illustrate the concepts and principles of *Introduction* in a way that would define how local flaps have influenced my plastic surgery practice. The keystone perforator island flap had become a trusted workhorse in my tool kit. So early in 2016 we produced *Defining Local Flaps: Clinical Applications and Methods.* Associate Professor Behan was recruited as the third author. The positive feedback from readers of this second book encouraged us to communicate with Springer's editors in Berlin, to produce a new book combining and expanding on the material in the forerunners. This is called *Simply Local Flaps.*

Our collective 100 years of plastic surgery experience is the cornerstone of this new book. How to share this knowledge, judgement and intuitive decision-making, when faced with reconstructive challenges, is the goal, and we hope that we may encourage the novice plastic surgeon and trainee to consider our method.

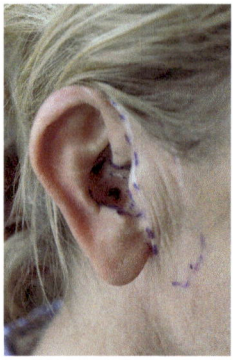 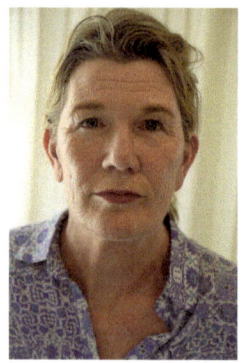

The 57-year-old woman (see figure, above) presented with an infiltrating basal cell carcinoma on the concha of her right ear. Does the surgeon choose the traditional reconstructive option of a mastoid 'revolving door' island flap for her repair, following wide excision of the tumour and underlying cartilage? She mentions that she would like to look a little more youthful in the face. Is there an option for using an inferiorly based preauricular transposition flap with a de-epithelialised bridging segment buried under the right earlobe? Is the serendipitous collision of reconstructive need and aesthetic desire an opportunity for innovative plastic surgery method?

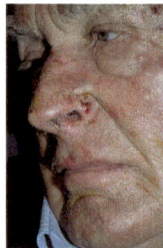 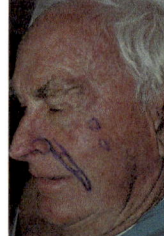 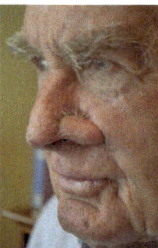 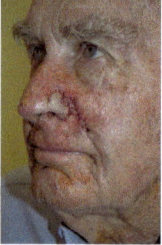 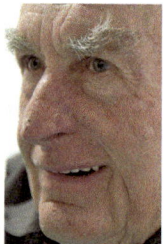

This 78-year-old man is shown before and 2 years after excision and staged reconstruction of the biopsy-proven squamous cell carcinoma on the left ala of his nose. He is a stoical hardworking person, but he needs to know what the management of this skin cancer requires.

How best to get a satisfactory aesthetic reconstruction, given the wide excision margins that are required? How to preserve the shape and contour of this unique bilateral nasal anatomical landmark? To use a graft or a local flap, with or without a cartilage graft for support? Can the nasal lining be safely preserved? If not, what is the best tissue to replace it with? These are the questions that we as experienced plastic surgeons think about automatically, after years of trial and error, successes and failures, happy and unhappy patients.

Plastic and reconstructive surgery is all about innovation.

New knowledge is only possible when thought is liberated from the grip of traditional tenets [1].

The basic principles of local flaps are a foundation for planning the repair. Proper plastic surgery method is not a cookbook approach. We believe that a good knowledge of basic reconstructive principles will enable the surgeon to create modifications of a standard flap, to fit the surgical problem (and not make the problem fit a standard flap).

Thanks to the willingness and permission for their images to be shared in this book, the patients have made possible an educational experience that may help the reader answer these questions for future patients and clinical challenges.

I hope so.

Epsom, Auckland, New Zealand   Michael F. Klaassen
January 2017

References

1. Matthews DN (1979) Gillies, Mastermind of Modern Plastic Surgery. British Journal of Plastic Surgery 32: 68–77

Acknowledgements

The authors wish to acknowledge the very generous support and encouragement of trustees of **The Sir William and Lady Lois Manchester Trust**, Judith Shea, David Ross, Tim Savage and the late Chris Horton.

The Manchester Trust is the legacy left by Sir William and Lady Lois Manchester for plastic surgery, the arts, education and the disadvantaged.

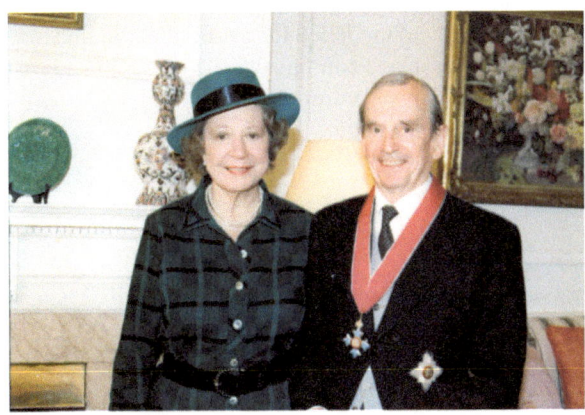

Lady Lois and Sir William Manchester

Sir William was an internationally renowned New Zealand plastic surgeon, with a particular reputation for the treatment of children with cleft lip and palate. He was highly regarded as a teacher. He was the Sir William Stevenson, Professor of Plastic Surgery at the University of Auckland and a popular visiting professor to many well-known plastic surgery centres around the world. He was the general secretary of the International Confederation of Plastic and Reconstructive Surgery. It was during this time that he rewrote the statutes and by-laws of the confederation, to restrict membership to fully trained plastic surgeons and improve the quality of training for young plastic surgeons in accredited training programmes. All of the authors knew and benefitted from Sir William's influence as a teacher of plastic surgery: Dr. Earle Brown as a trainee in Auckland, Dr. Felix Behan as a fellow in London and Dr. Michael Klaassen as a trainee when Sir William had retired but regularly visited the Middlemore Hospital Plastic Surgery Unit. Lady Lois was an internationally acclaimed interior designer and successful businesswoman. She was very supportive of her husband in his work and contributed equally to their charitable trust. She had a gracious personality and was always generous in her support for the staff of the Plastic Surgery Unit at Middlemore Hospital and their families.

Special thanks go to the following:

Mrs. Val Grey (graphic designer), formerly of the University of Auckland, who was the graphic designer and layout expert for the two forerunners of this book.

Dr. Swee Tan (ONZM, MBBS, PhD, FRACS) for providing Fig. 9.27 and for his foreword. Dr. Tan has also been a monolithic supporter for this project, with his advice, multiple reviews of the chapters and literary skills.

Dr. Peter Charlesworth (FRACS) for his contribution to the paragraphs about Dr. Michael Flint's circle method for planning the best incisions in the relaxed skin tension lines.

All the patients who kindly gave permission to Dr. Michael Klaassen for their clinical images to be used in the following pages.

Robbie Turner of London who modelled for the Flint circle illustrations.

Tania Hoang of Sydney for image editing advice.

Diana Savoy for proofreading and editing.

Our wives for their continuing support.

Contents

Part I   Fundamentals

1   Introduction   3
   What Are Local Flaps?   6
   Classification of Local Flaps   7
   Planning a Local Flap   8
   Aesthetic Subunit Principle   8
   Scar Considerations   8
   Flint's Circle Technique for Determining the Optimum Scar Lines   10
   Anatomical Landmarks   11
   Sources of Spare Skin on the Face of Good Donor Sites
   for Skin Flaps   11
   References   12

2   Getting Started: Planning and Drawing   15
   Planning with Flint's Circles   19
   References   20

3   Technical Tips for Local Flap Surgery   21
   Documentation   21
   Local Anaesthesia   21
   Sterile Technique   22
   Standard Surgical Instruments   23
   Gentle Tissue Handling   25
   Suture Without Tension   25
   Photograph and Measure Everything for the Record, Especially
   Complications of Treatment   26
   Precise Surgical Dissection   26
   Designing a Local Flap to Avoid Tension in Hand Wound Defects   29
   Managing Patients on Aspirin and Anticoagulants   29
   References   29

Part II Traditional Local Flaps

4 Elliptical Excision and Sliding Flap Repair   33
   Modifications of the Ellipse   34
   Crescentic Ellipse   36
   Asymmetrical Ellipse   36
   Wedge Excision.   37
   M-plasty   38
   Crown Excision.   39
   Modifications of the Wedge Excision   40
   Dog-ears   42
   Summary.   43
   References.   43

5 Advancement Flaps.   45
   Single Pedicle Advancement Flaps.   46
   Dorsal Nasal Flap   47
   Mucosal Advancement Flap   48
   Double Advancement Flap   50
      Biwinged Flap.   50
   Perialar Crescentic Advancement Flaps   52
   Double Advancement Flaps   53
      H-plasty.   53
      Flaps Involving V-Y Advancement   54
   Nasalis Flap.   55
   Upper Lip Case   56
   Sigmoid Oblique Advancement Flap   57
   Double V-Y Flaps   59
      Kite Flaps   59
   V-Y Technique for Closing Surgical Wounds.   60
   The V-Y Technique for Releasing Scar Contractures   60
   Y-V Advancement.   61
   Multiple Y-V Advancement Flaps.   62
   Bipedicle Advancement Flap   63
   References.   63

6 Rotation Flaps   65
   Rotation Flap to Scalp.   67
   Rotation Flap Requiring a Skin Graft to Repair Flap Donor Site.   68
      Rotation Flap in the Temporal Area   68
      Rotation Flap for Buttock Defects   69
      Rotation Flaps on the Face   69
      Bilateral Rotation Flaps for Repairing Lower Lip   71
      Neurovascular Cheek and Lip Flaps.   71
      Modifications of the Rotation Flap.   72
      Subtotal Forehead Flap.   73
   References.   75

7 Interpolated Flaps.   77
   Paramedian Forehead Flap   78
   Interpolated Flap with Buried Pedicle   80
   Subcutaneous Pedicle Flaps on Other Parts of the Face   81
   Vascular Island Flaps   82
   Serendipity Flap   82
   The Bipedicle Upper Eyelid Flap   83
   References.   84

8 Transposition Flaps.   85
   Postauricular Flap (Inferiorly Based)   87
   Postauricular Flap (Superiorly Based) to the Ear   88
   Nasolabial Flap (Inferiorly Based)   89
   Nasolabial Flap (Superiorly Based)   90
   Dorsal Nasoaxial Flap.   92
   Glabellar Flap   92
   Lower Eyelid Flap.   93
   Rhomboid Flap   95
   Square Peg in a Round Hole   98
   Dufourmental Flap   101
   Comparison of the Rhombic and Dufourmental Flaps   102
   Swing-Slide Plasty   103
   Banner Flap.   106
   Hatchet Flap or V-Y-S Closure for a Circular Defect   107
   References.   107

9 Triangular Flaps That Transpose, Advance and Interdigitate   109
   Z-Plasty.   109
   Planning a Scar Revision on the Face.   116
   Planning Z-Plasties in Three Dimensions.   117
   Notching of the Lip.   117
   Bridle Scar   117
   Congenital Ring Constriction   118
   Modifying the Z-Plasty Flaps   119
   Tetrahedral Z-Plasty   119
   Finger Web   120
   Asymmetrical Z-Plasty.   121
   Altering Angle Size.   121
   The Jumping Man Flap.   123
   Use of Z-Plasty in Flap Repairs   123
   The Double Z to Rhomboid Plasty   125
   Rhomboid to W-Plasty   125
   Triangular Flaps that Advance and Interdigitate.   127
      W-Plasty   127
   The Effects of a W-Plasty   128
   References.   128

10   **Hinge Flaps** 129
     Cross Finger Flap 133
     References... 133

11   **Recommended Traditional Local Flaps** 135
     Rotation Scalp Flap.. 135
     Paramedian Forehead Flap 136
     Biwinged Excision/Sliding Advancement Flaps.................. 136
     Sigmoid Oblique Advancement Flap 137
     Nasolabial Flap (Superiorly Based) 137
     Dorsal Nasoaxial Flap.. 137
     Glabellar Flap 138
     Transposition Cheek Flap 138
     Karapandzic Flaps.. 139
     Dorsal Hand Flap 139
     References... 140

Part III   Modern Local Flaps

12   **Keystone Flap Concepts** 143
     Anatomy and Physiology 143
     Flap Design.. 144
     Surgical Technique for Keystone Flap 145
     References... 146

13   **Favoured Keystone Flap Applications**....................... 147
     Cheek 147
     Lateral Nose 149
     Upper Lip 149
     Forehead, Temple and Scalp................................... 150
     Neck 152
     Shoulder 153
     Trunk.. 154
     Lower Limb... 156
     Hand 157
     Foot... 159

14   **Combination Flaps** 161
     Keystone Advancement + Chin Rotation Flaps 161
     Cervicofacial Rotation + Glabellar Transposition Flaps....... 162
     Forehead Interpolated Flap + Cheek Rotation
     Flap + Lip Switch Flap....................................... 162
     Combination Keystone Flaps from Cervical and Cheek Regions... 163

Part IV Judgement, Decision-making and Experience

15 Where Skin Grafts Are Better 167
    Scalp 167
    Frontal Region 168
    Nose 169
    The Upper Lip. 171

16 Aesthetica. 173
    Bilateral Preauricular Skin Grafts. 173
    Facelift flaps 175
        Type I: Mini Preauricular Facelift Flaps. 175
        Type 2: Moderate Preauricular Facelift Flap 176
        Type 3: Extended Facelift Flap. 177
    References. 178

17 Complications: Their Management and Prevention 179
    Haematoma. 179
    Venous Ischaemia 180
    Radiation Necrosis 181
    Secondary Viral Infection 182
    Hypertrophic Scars 183
    Ectropion Deformity. 184
    Oncological Issues 185
    Risk Awareness and Consent 185

18 How to Think Like a Plastic Surgeon 187
    Case A. 187
    Case B. 190

Appendix 195
    Part V 195
        Other Resources Considered for this Book but not Formally
        Referenced 195

Glossary 197

Index. 199

About the Authors

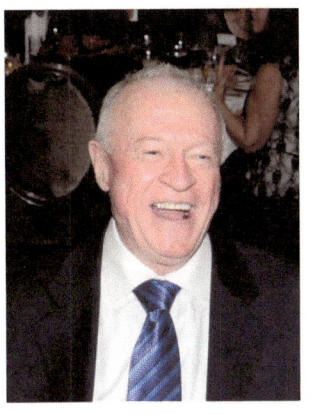

Felix Behan is a former associate professor of plastic surgery in Melbourne, Australia. Born in Queensland, he graduated in medicine from the University of Queensland in 1964. He trained in plastic surgery in Melbourne under Sir Benjamin Rank (a pupil of Gillies, McIndoe and Mowlem) and gained his FRACS in 1970. He then headed for London, England where he gained an FRCS in 1971, having worked as a senior registrar at St. George's Hospital (Westminster) and The Royal Marsden Hospital, Fulham. Concurrently he was a Nuffield research fellow at RCS England, investigating the vascularity of tissue flaps. He returned to Melbourne to be Sir Benjamin's aide-de-camp and worked as a consultant plastic surgeon at Peter MacCallum Cancer Centre and the Western Hospital, Melbourne, where he was the clinical chief of plastic, reconstructive and hand surgery for many years. He is best known as the pioneer of the keystone perforator island flap and has published extensively on this workhorse loco-regional flap.

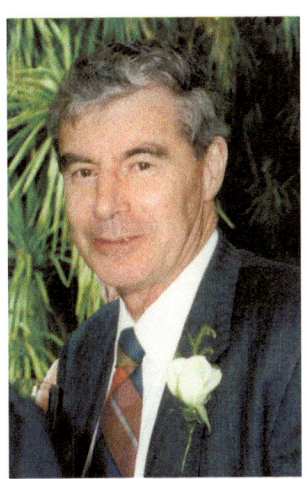

Earle Brown is a graduate of Otago University with MBChB in 1960. He completed his training in general surgery in Auckland and the UK, obtaining the FRCS.

His initial plastic surgery training was at Middlemore Hospital under the tutelage of Sir William Manchester and Dr. John Williams. Sir William had been a pupil of Gillies, McIndoe and Mowlem during WWII. Dr. Brown undertook further plastic surgery training as a registrar and senior registrar at Canniesburn Hospital in Glasgow.

He returned to the Plastic Surgery Unit at Middlemore Hospital in 1970, obtained FRACS in plastic surgery and was appointed consultant plastic surgeon from 1970 to 2005. He was clinical head of the department from 1990 to 1997 and clinical director of surgery from 1997 to 2002. During the 1980s, he gathered a large collection of copied journal and textbook articles on local flaps. These were distributed to the registrars in training. These notes were later edited and updated by Dr. Michael Klaassen and formed the basis of *Introduction to Local Flaps: A Surgeon's Handbook*, published in 2011. *Defining Local Flaps: Clinical Applications and Methods*, published in 2016, was another collaboration with Drs. Klaassen and Behan.

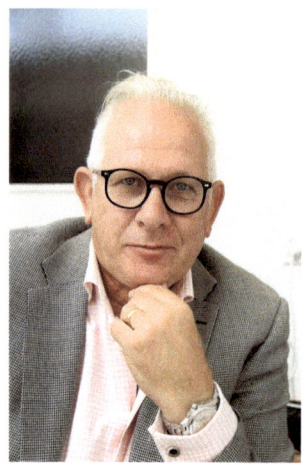

Michael Klaassen graduated with an MBChB from Otago University in 1980 and qualified as a plastic surgeon in 1990 after completing his training at Middlemore and Waikato Hospitals in New Zealand. Dr. Earle Brown was his original mentor in plastic and reconstructive surgery in 1987. Together they wrote *Introduction to Local Flaps: A Surgeon's Handbook* in 2011, whilst he was director of surgical skills at the University of Auckland. In 2016, they wrote *Defining Local Flaps: Clinical Applications and Methods* and included the work and concepts of Associate Professor Felix Behan from Melbourne, Australia. Dr. Klaassen lives in Auckland but in the last 4 years has developed a provincial plastic surgery practice that extends from Pukekohe to Hamilton, the Bay of Plenty and Gisborne, New Zealand.

Part I

Fundamentals

Chapter 1: Introduction

The teaching philosophy and clinical experience behind the motivation to create another book on Local Flaps.

Chapter 2: Getting Started: Drawing and Planning

How best to begin to understand the clinical planning and design of local flaps, with an emphasis on visualization, artistic skills and learning to draw.

Chapter 3: Technical Tips for Local Flap Surgery

Over the years we have developed a number of methods for enabling the efficient and safe practice of plastic surgery. We believe these are worth sharing.

Introduction

1

Over the past 7 years, we have organised coaching courses for senior plastic surgery trainees preparing for their final fellowship examination. Many of the principles that we champion from Paré, Gillies [1], McIndoe [2], Millard [3] and Manchester [4] are illustrated in the definition, design and application of local flaps for plastic surgical repair/reconstruction.

The *key principles* include:

1. Diagnose before you treat.
2. Make a plan and a pattern.
3. Make a record.
4. The lifeboat.
5. Treat the primary defect first.
6. Losses must be replaced in kind.
7. Never let routine method become your master.
8. The aftercare is as important as the planning.
    (*Sir Harold Gillies*)
9. Connection with your patient equals confident patient.
    (*Sir Archibald McIndoe*)
10. Know the 'ideal' beautiful normal.
11. Teaching our specialty is its best legacy.
    (*Dr. Ralph Millard Jr.*)
12. Is there tissue missing or displaced?
13. How much and what tissue is missing?
14. Perfection is only just good enough.
    (*Sir William Manchester*)

It is the evolution of these courses with Dr. Earle Brown, Dr. Michael Leung (Melbourne) and Dr. Mark Moore (Adelaide), which has motivated us to produce reading and resource material, which will be useful before, during and well after the courses, when participants are face-to-face with real patients and real repair/reconstructive challenges.

© Springer International Publishing AG 2018
M.F. Klaassen et al., *Simply Local Flaps*,
https://doi.org/10.1007/978-3-319-59400-2_1

All three authors have participated in practical flap teaching courses for junior plastic surgical trainees. These courses have included some theory but have concentrated on the practice of surgery, planning and raising local flaps on pig skin.

The lead author, with the support of Interplast Australia and New Zealand, has for some years organised and taught flap courses to Pacific Island surgeons and trainees as part of their Continuing Surgical Education [5].

Simply Local Flaps evolved out of the initial *Introduction to Local Flaps* [6] and the subsequent *Defining Local Flaps* [7]. The earlier texts were designed to be read together so it seemed logical to combine and expand them into a single book with added material.

Fig. 1.1 Dr. Earle Brown FRACS, teaching local flaps at the inaugural introduction to local flaps workshop (2013)

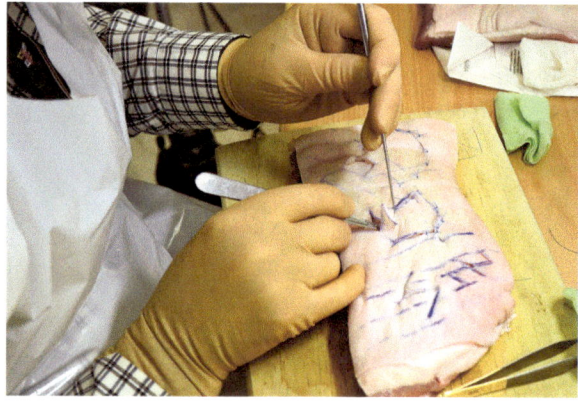

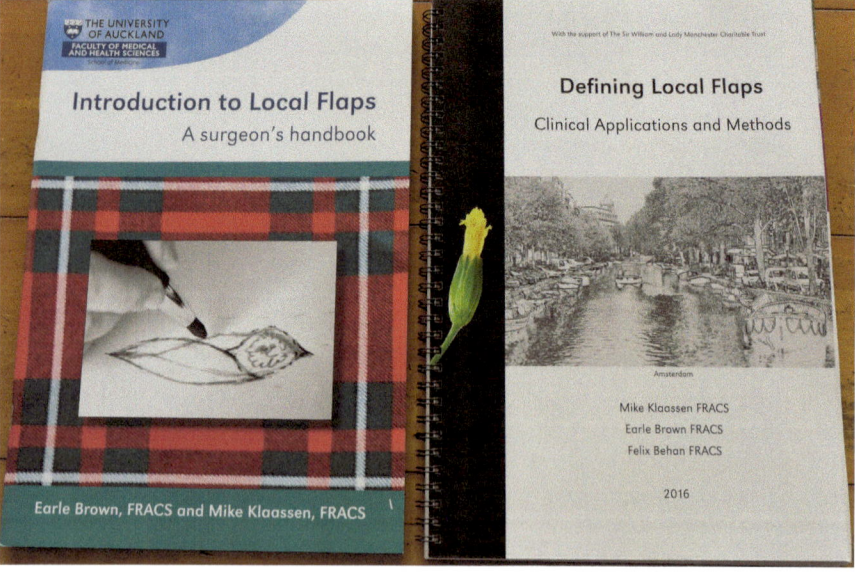

Fig. 1.2 Introduction and defining local flaps (the forerunners)

Simply Local Flaps is an instructional atlas based on the theory and principles of plastic surgery combined with extensive clinical experience. The clinical cases (except Figure 9.27) are all from the lead author's plastic surgical practice and are flaps he has used for cutaneous defects over the last 10 years.

Where possible, the latest photograph illustrating the healed and stable result is included.

Although local flaps are the focus, a chapter is dedicated to clinical cases, where the authors believe a *skin graft (either split, full thickness or composite)* is a superior reconstructive option.

The rest of the *introduction* summarises the important principles pertaining to local flaps, followed by chapters on *getting started, design and planning* and *technical tips for local flap surgery.*

Traditional local flaps and the theory and principles of keystone perforator island flaps are described in separate Parts.

Clinical cases with *surgical methods* are then described with illustrations and description. The final chapters include *scar therapy* and *how to manage complications*, when they occur. The flap complications are again all from the lead author's practice and have been a challenge that has required careful thought and action. Without doubt, every surgeon will have to face and deal with complications. It is how to recognise them early, manage them proactively and support your patient through this challenging and difficult period that defines a complete surgeon. This, in our experience, will maintain understanding and loyalty from your patient. This chapter was the most difficult to write, because of the memories, but may even be the most important chapter of the book. We all forget our successes, but never our failures—they will haunt you for the period of your career. But with an open and attentive mind, you will learn from them.

Finally, in an effort to summarise the way principles, clinical judgment, experience and local flap selection are integrated as a whole, we have added a chapter on *How to think like a plastic surgeon.* These are two clinical cases, presenting to the lead author, with discussion and comment from the other authors. The questions and answers posed, combined with the surgical plan, staged reconstruction and final results will hopefully add to the educational value of this book.

Where appropriate, we mention the historical relevance and origins of plastic surgery methods. 'We are like dwarfs sitting on the shoulders of giants' as John of Salisbury (1120–1180) once stated. Although less popular in this modern

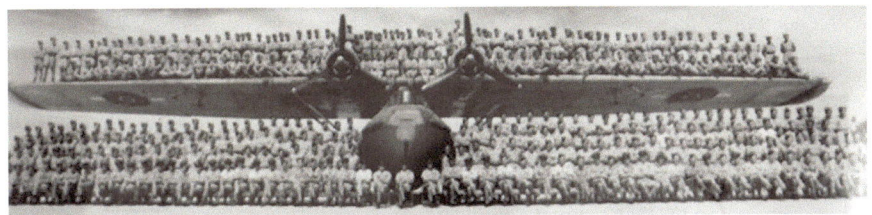

Fig. 1.3 '… on the shoulders of giants.' RNZAF No. 6 Squadron & Seacat Flying Boat (1944)—courtesy of the late Keith Challon RIP (Whakatane, NZ)

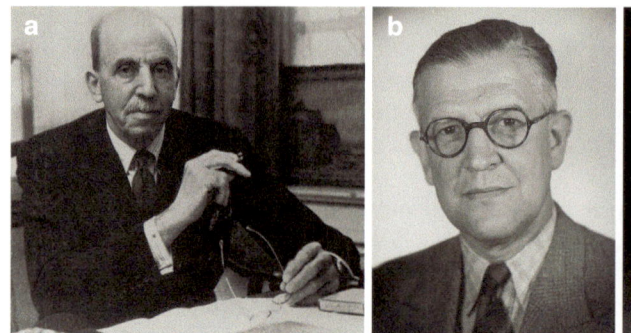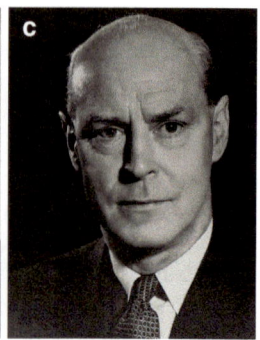

Fig. 1.4 Sir Harold Gillies, Sir Archibald McIndoe, Dr. Rainsford Mowlem

competitive world, the recognition and acknowledgement of the early pioneers is important in our view.

Three of the great pioneers are illustrated above:

During their professional lives, the authors have spent much time treating skin tumours. These are a consequence of high ultraviolet radiation, in white-skinned people of European origin and the 'beach' culture in our countries of New Zealand and Australia. Whilst preventative programmes are in place to reduce our sun exposure, we are still seeing large numbers of patients, with solar damage to their skin.

The treatment of these skin tumours is primarily by surgery. Many of these lesions can be treated by a simple elliptical excision and the defect closed directly. For larger lesions, longer or wider elliptical excisions are required, until the stage is reached where it is not possible to oppose skin edges. This is where a local flap has to be considered.

What Are Local Flaps?

Local flaps are units of skin and subcutaneous tissue, planned and raised adjacent to the wound and transferred in such a way to make good the defect, without creating a secondary defect.

Flaps differ from skin grafts, in having an intact blood supply *at all times*.

The flap is transferred from the donor site to the recipient site whilst maintaining its own blood supply.

The word 'flap' originated allegedly from the sixteenth-century Dutch word *FLAPPE*, which referred to *anything that hung broad and loose, fastened only by one side.*

Whilst the term flap is part of the plastic surgical nomenclature, we were unable to discover when it was first used in a surgical context. Flap repairs are an integral part of plastic and reconstructive surgery and can vary in tissue composition and size, depending on the surgical defect to be repaired.

Classification of Local Flaps

Local flaps can be classified according to:

1. Their method of transfer
2. Blood supply
3. Composition
4. Shape of the wound

There are many ways of classifying all types of flap repair in plastic surgery.

We favour the system proposed by Professor David Tolhurst [8], where he identifies the various kinds of flap, both local and regional. He refers to this system as the *atomic classification*, where he compares all flap repairs with the nucleus and electron shells of an atom. The nucleus lists the tissue components of flaps and the outer shell system lists the various characteristics of the flaps. This is illustrated in Fig. 1.5.

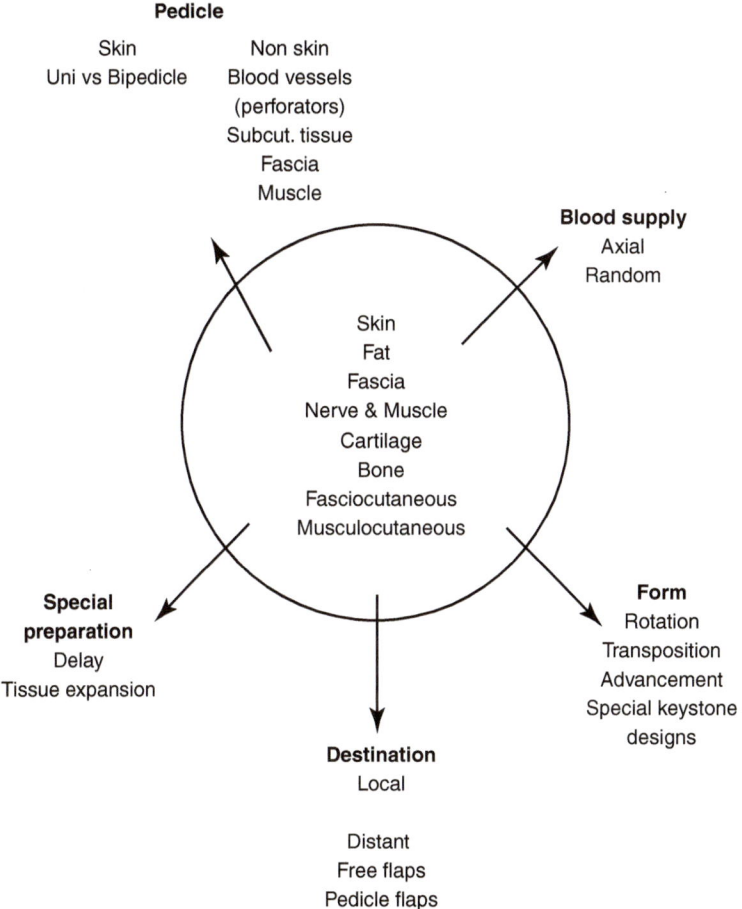

Fig. 1.5 The atomic system for classification of flaps by David Tolhurst (with his express permission)

In the Part II of this book, we use traditional methods, where local flaps are classified according to the way they are moved into the surgical defect.

In Part III, we introduce the keystone flap and illustrate its versatility.

In general terms, the classification of local flaps is defined by describing their method of transfer. This is either by *advancement, movement of the flap around a pivot point or a combination of these.*

Planning a Local Flap

With experience, many local flaps can be mentally visualised. Others, however, require careful consideration and 'planning in reverse' using oiled silk or similar material before proceeding with the operation. This empirical approach to planning is based on the surgeon's experience. The introduction of local flaps, designed with mathematical precision and detailed analysis of skin biomechanics following transfer, have made flap planning more precise. The pioneer in this field was Dr. A. A. Limberg from Leningrad, whose original 1946 monograph on *The Mathematical Basis of Local Plastic Procedures on the Human Body Surface* was translated by Dr. S. Anthony Wolfe in 1984 [9]. Dr. Earle Brown has generously given me his copy.

One still has to be aware of the important factors in planning, which include:

1. Appreciation of where there is skin tension and where there is spare skin
2. Possible displacement of anatomical landmarks
3. Possible trapdoor deformity
4. Scar orientation

The flap donor site should be considered in any repair. Dieffenbach [10] succinctly referred to this: .... *It is of equal importance with the restoration of the lost part to preserve the existing one. Surgeons are not warranted in causing a considerable deformity in one place, in order to cover a defect in another ...*

Aesthetic Subunit Principle

As pioneered by Drs. Gary Burget and Fred Menick [11], the anatomical nasal aesthetic subunit principle should be respected and followed for the achievement of aesthetic reconstruction to give the best results. If the defect is 50% or more of the aesthetic unit, excise the whole unit and reconstruct/repair it.

Scar Considerations

All surgery and wounding produces scars, which are permanent and characterised by a predictable physiologic response: healing. Scar appearance is the key issue for the patient, especially when involving the face. Expectation and psychosocial issues determine that the face is of particular concern for patients, young and old.

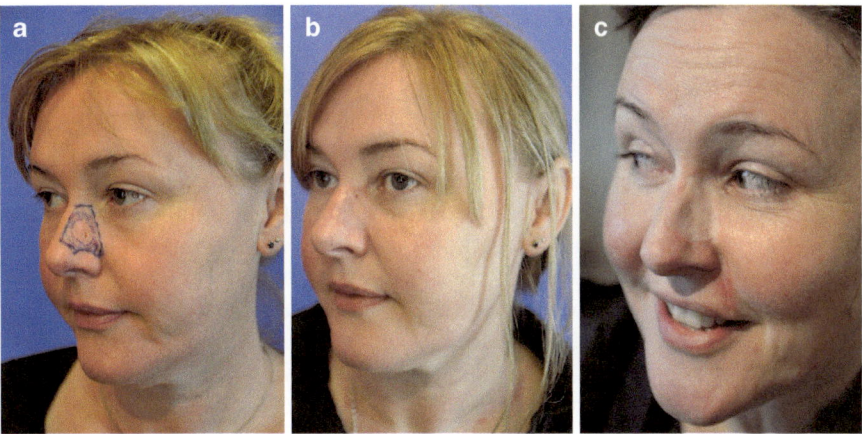

Fig. 1.6 Aesthetic subunit principle of repair applied with a full thickness supraclavicular skin graft to the left nasal sidewall in a 43-year-old woman with sclerosing BCC (**a**), 6 weeks (**b**) and 2 years (**c**) after surgery

It is helpful to communicate to the patient simple facts about the natural progress and time frame of various scars. These include the important role of postoperative care, prevention of bad scars and scar revision when required. Scar improvement is linked to the ability to change the width of the scar, its direction and configuration.

Scar revision techniques include broken line camouflage methods (Deckling) and lengthening methods (multiple Z-plasties and W-plasties). Photographic analysis and documentation are essential concepts in scar therapy.

As a principle, one of the goals of local flap surgery should be the avoidance of unsightly and bad scars (hypertrophic/keloid). The timeless principles of Gillies, developed during the First World War and the pre-antibiotic era, are worth remembering: gentle atraumatic tissue handling with skin hooks rather than crushing tissue forceps, precise and accurate approximation of soft tissue margins without tension and reduction and stabilisation of the underlying bony structures.

In the modern world, the concepts of Albert F. Borges for optimizing the quality of incisional scars are legendary [12]. He taught us to camouflage a scar, by having its direction follow the *relaxed skin tension lines (RSTLs)*, as much as possible. He said *Never incise at right angles to the relaxed skin tension lines*. Relaxed skin tension lines are those tension lines that follow the furrows formed, when the skin is relaxed. They are not visible features of the skin, such as wrinkle lines, but can be found by pinching the skin and observing the furrows and ridges that are formed.

Fortunately, the RSTLs are the same in all persons. 'Langer's lines' are important only from a historical perspective (see Flint's circle technique). They represent the skin tension lines in rigor mortis. RSTLs and Langer's lines do not correspond in many areas of the body.

It is possible to design local flaps with the RSTLs in mind.

Flint's Circle Technique for Determining the Optimum Scar Lines

Dr Michael Flint, a British-trained plastic surgeon and surgical researcher in the Department of Surgery, School of Medicine, University of Auckland, studied wound healing and further elucidated and extended the findings of Langer, Cox and others [13, 14, 15]. In 1979 [16], he described his technique for determining the best incision lines for acceptable scarring: *The circle technique* (Flint's circles). Serendipitously he observed that imprinted circles of 1–2 cm diameter, using a simple rubber stamp, on the trunk and limbs of a human subject in the flexed foetal position, deformed into ellipses when the subject resumed the anatomical unflexed position. The long axes of these ellipses are aligned with the direction of skin tension. Dr. Tom Gibson from Glasgow and Canniesburn Hospital referred to the lines of cleavage as the lines of minimal extensibility (LME). The LME run at right angles to the direction of maximum extensibility (LMxE). Subsequently, Flint used his simple rubber stamps and circle technique in surgical practice to determine the direction of skin tension (LME) and therefore the relaxed skin tension lines (RSTLs) for optimal scarring.

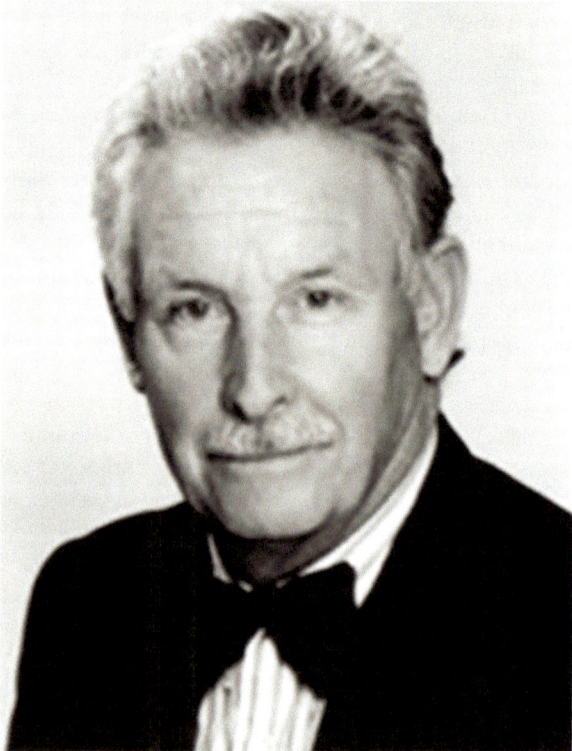

Fig. 1.7 Dr. Michael Flint

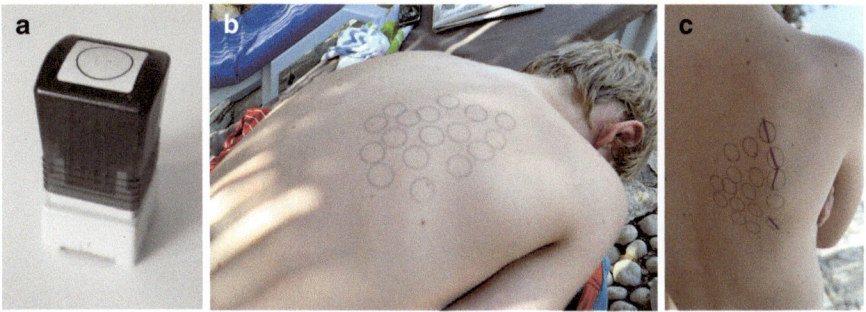

Fig. 1.8 The use of the Flint circle technique. These photos show the circular stamp (**a**) and its use on the back of a 12-year-old boy, in the flexed (**b**) and unflexed position (**c**) (Thanks to Robbie Turner of London, who modelled for this demonstration)

As well as determining the ideal line of surgical incision, the circles also warn of potential wound closure difficulties. If there is no change in the shape of the circle (no elliptical deformation), this indicates that the tensional forces are equal in all directions. There will be little potential for the skin to stretch and a local flap or graft repair may be.

Anatomical Landmarks

In the head and neck, there are some standard landmarks, which should not be moved or distorted by the proposed local flap surgery [17].

These include:

1. Anterior hairline
2. Eyebrows
3. Eyelids and canthi
4. Nasal tip and alae
5. Perialar cheek groove
6. Earlobes
7. Philtrum
8. Vermillion
9. Oral commissure

Sources of Spare Skin on the Face of Good Donor Sites for Skin Flaps

Forehead—this can be fairly tight, but there is always some skin laxity in the glabellar region (V-Y glabellar flap).
Cheek—especially the nasolabial folds and preauricular regions.
Neck—cervical and mandibular regions, including the jowls.
Temple—questionable in our experience.

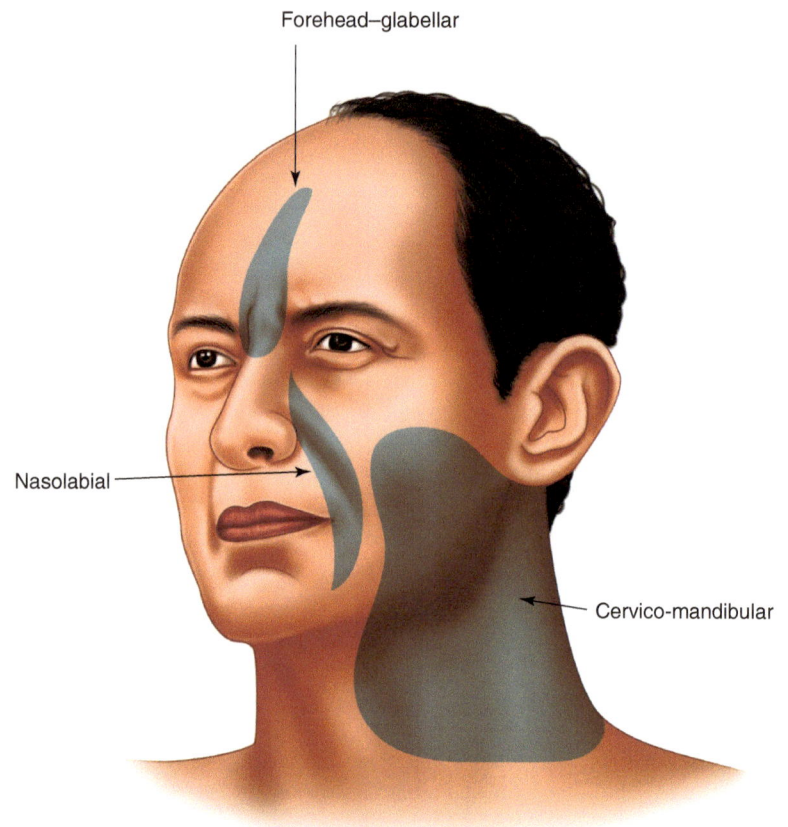

Fig. 1.9 Areas of spare skin (from McGregor's Fundamental Techniques of Plastic Surgery (1989, 8th edition) [17]

References

1. Gillies HD (1920) Plastic surgery of the face. Henry Frowde/Oxford University Press, London
2. McIndoe AH (1983), Total reconstruction of the burned face. The Bradshaw Lecture 1958. Br. J Plast Surg 36(4):410–420.
3. Millard DR (1986) Principlization of plastic surgery. Lippincott Williams & Wilkins, Baltimore
4. Manchester WM. The repair of double cleft lip as part of integrated program. Plast. Reconstr Surg. 1970;45: 205. + Manchester Lecture Notes (1951) in Manchester Archives (Held by E. Brown FRACS).
5. Brown E, Klaassen M (2011) Introduction to local flaps: a surgeon's handbook. University of Auckland, School of Medicine, Auckland
6. Klaassen M, Brown E, Behan FC. Defining local flaps: clinical applications and methods. Self published. 2016.
7. Klaassen M, Thomson S (2014) Flap reference handbook. Interplast, East Melbourne
8. Tolhurst DE. Fasciocutaneous flaps (Thesis for PhD), Drukkeru Pasmans B.V., 's- Gravenhage. 1988.

9. Limberg A.A. (1946), Planirovanye mestnoplasticheskikh operatsii na poverkhnosti tela—The planning of local plastic operations of the body surface—Theory and practice. (Translated by S. Anthony Wolfe MD, 1984). Lexington: Collamore Press.
10. Dieffenbach JF (1794–1847) As quoted by Hayes H. in An anthology of plastic surgery, vol 1986. Aspen, Rockville
11. Burget G, Menick F (1994) Aesthetic reconstruction of the nose. St. Mosby, Louis
12. Borges AF, Alexander JE (1962) Relaxed skin tension lines Z-plasties on scars and fusiform excision of lesions. Br J Plast Surg 15:242–254
13. Dupuytren G (1836) Uber die Verletzungen durch Kriegswaffen. Aus d, Franz
14. Langer C. 1861. "Zur Anatomie und Physiologie der Haut. Über die Spaltbarkeit der Cutis". Sitzungsbericht der Mathematisch-naturwissenschaftlichen Classe der Wiener Kaiserlichen Academie der Wissenschaften Abt. 44 (Br. J Plast Surg. 31(1):3–8, 1978, (translation of original): 'On the anatomy and physiology of the skin.' Online version: DOI.10.1016/0007-1226(78)90003-6
15. Cox HT (1941) The Cleavage Lines of the Skin. Br J Surg 29:234
16. Flint M. H. (1979), The Development of the Circle Technique for Determining the Optimum Line of Tumour Excision. Aust. N.Z. J. Surg. Vol. 49 (6), 690–696. Online version: DOI.10.1111/j.1445-2197.tb0649.x
17. McGregor IA (1989) Fundamental techniques of plastic surgery, 8th edn. Churchill Livingstone, Edinburgh

Check for
updates

Getting Started: Planning and Drawing

2

The wide range of local flaps described in this book may seem overwhelming to the novice. The best approach initially is to familiarize yourself with the classification of local flaps and their broad defining groups. The understanding of how the individual local flaps either advance, transpose, rotate around a pivot point or move by a combination of rotation and advancement is essential. With experience, you will begin to appreciate which flaps work best in different anatomical regions.

Drawing and visualizing what you are planning to do is an essential plastic surgical skill. Not everyone is a natural artist, but with some simple tips and practice, you can improve your drawing skills quite quickly. One approach is to take a digital image and then make a simple line drawing of the image. Onto this, you can outline the edge of the tumour/wound, the resection margins/debridement and the options for local flap repair. A full thickness skin graft may be an alternative repair option or you could let the wound heal by secondary intention (this is commonly the case with forehead flap donor sites).

© Springer International Publishing AG 2018

M.F. Klaassen et al., *Simply Local Flaps*,

https://doi.org/10.1007/978-3-319-59400-2_2

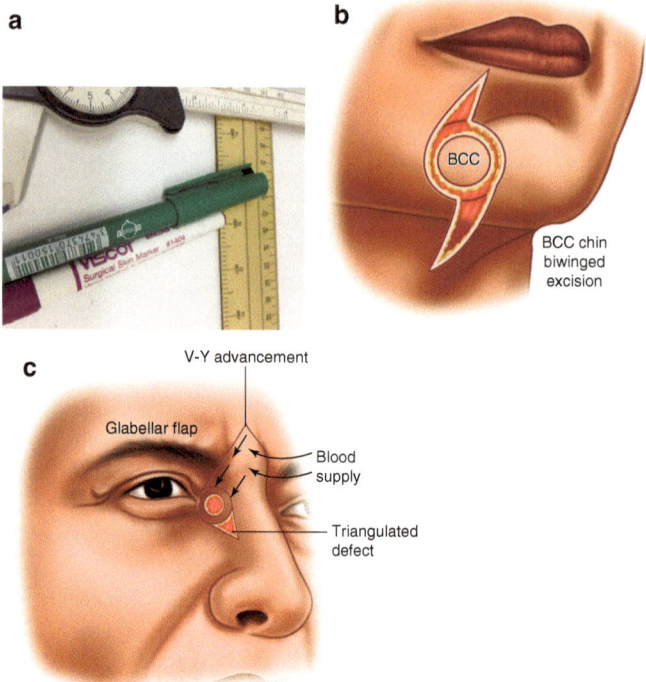

Fig. 2.1 Simple drawing tools (**a**), plan for biwinged excision large BCC on the chin (**b**) and glabellar V-Y transposition/advancement flap for similar infiltrating BCC right medial canthus (**c**). 5 mm margins of resection and triangulation of the medial canthal defect. Blood supply from the left paranasal contralateral side. A full thickness preauricular skin graft is a good alternative

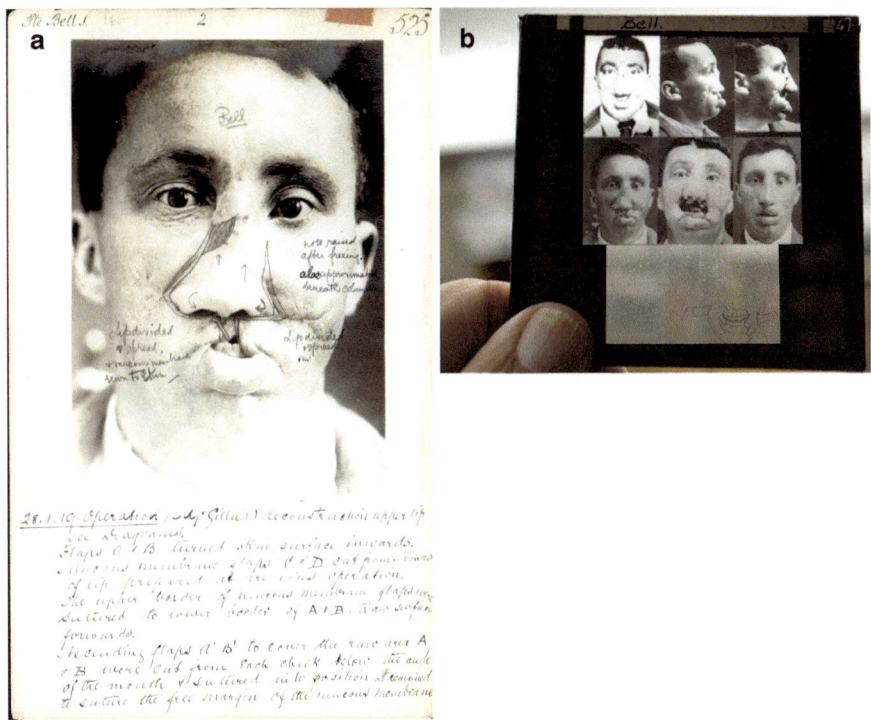

Fig. 2.2 'Make a plan and a pattern'—surgical plan and drawings of Captain Harold Gillies FRCS, Queen's Hospital, Sidcup, Kent (1919) for Private Bell, referred to him by Dr. Charles Valadier from France, following gunshot injury to midface. Glass slide collection shows final result circa 1920. Images courtesy of Dr. Andrew Bamji (former rheumatologist and Gillies Archivist at Sidcup Hospital, Kent, UK and from the Archives of The Royal College of Surgeons of England)

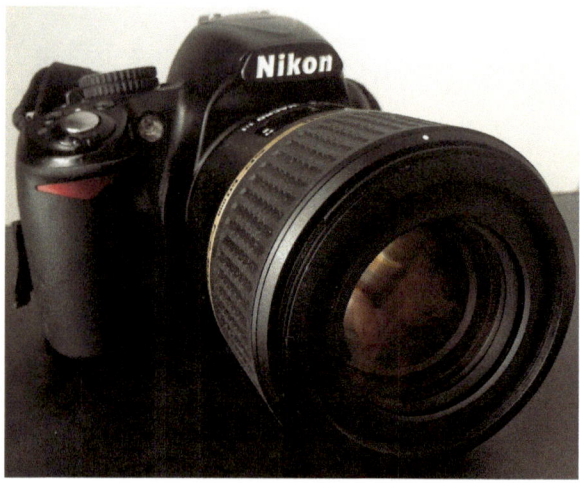

Fig. 2.3 My current camera, Nikon D3100 with a 60 mm F/2 Tamron macro lens. A number of cameras are useful. Woodrow Wilson of www.clinicalimaging.com.au recommends consumer grade DSLR with lens between 60 and 100 mm

Fig. 2.4 Plan for resection and reconstruction of a large infiltrating BCC of the lateral canthal/eyelids periorbital region in a 91-year-old gentleman. Large right lateral periorbital defect anticipated after wide margins of excision, so combination of local flaps planned (see result in Chap. 18)

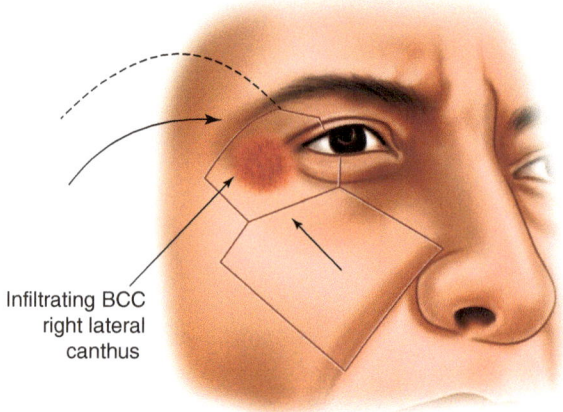

Infiltrating BCC
right lateral
canthus

Planning with Flint's Circles

These are particularly useful on the trunk and limbs.

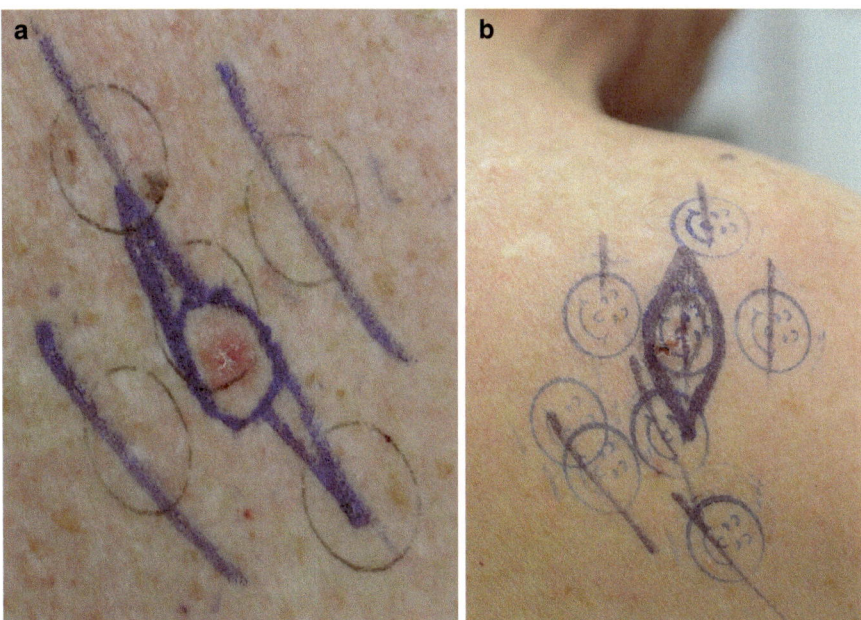

Fig. 2.5 (**a, b**) Flint's circles changed to ovoid shape to reveal the Relaxed Skin Tension Lines (RSTL) for wide excision of nodular BCC on the right scapular region of a 77-year-old woman. Initial stamps applied with the patient bent over in the flexed foetal position to put the back skin under tension (**a**). Similar Flint's circles for a 50-year-old man with BCC same region (**b**)

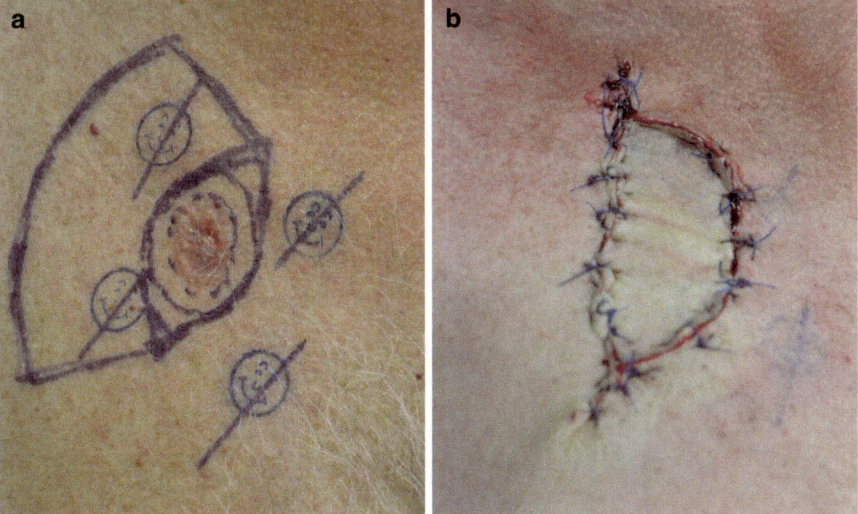

Fig. 2.6 Flint's circles used to plan the optimum scar lines for the wide excision of an infiltrating BCC on the presternum of a 65-year-old man and repair with a keystone perforator island local flap

References

1. Wilson W. Photo tips. Clinical Imaging Australia Pty Ltd. 2016. https://www.clinicalimaging.com.au.
2. Flint MH (1979) The development of the circle technique for determining the optimum line of tumour excision. Aust. N.Z. J. Surg 49(6):690–696. doi:10.1111/j.1445-2197.tb0649.x

Technical Tips for Local Flap Surgery

3

Preparedness, organisation and teamwork are essential for your surgical facility, whether it be office based or hospital based. The following are the important facts and systems developed over more than 26 years for the lead author's plastic surgery practice.

Documentation

This and patient safety are paramount. Completion of documentation of informed consent, operative notes and post-operative instructions is mandatory. Excised specimens should contain an orientation suture, be correctly labelled and be accompanied by clinical information for the Histo-pathologist. This is essential particularly if practicing from a number of clinics in provincial centres as I now do.

Local Anaesthesia

I use a combination of short-acting 1% lignocaine with adrenaline and long-acting 0.75% ropivacaine, which has an associated vasoconstriction effect. These are both from the amino amide group of local anaesthetic drugs [1].

The *safe doses* are:

Lignocaine	Plain (3–4 mg/kg) + adrenaline (5–7 mg/kg)
Quick acting with medium duration	
Naropin (ropivacaine)	Plain (3–4 mg/kg) + adrenaline (3–4 mg/kg)
Medium time for action but long duration	

Marcaine, another amino amide is the most toxic of all local anaesthetic drugs. Cardiotoxicity from overdose is almost always fatal, and I do not use it, ever.

After infiltrating the field of surgery with a safe dosage of local anaesthetic, *I wait at least 10–15 min* before commencing surgery. During this time I complete documentation, operative records and photographic archiving.

Sterile Technique

Asepsis and universal precautions are followed according to standard intraoperative protocols, but for minor surgery, I do not wear a mask or hat.

I frequently use loupe magnification (Designs for Visions 2.5×) or the Dr. Kim headlight (South Korea) with its 1.5× magnification lens system.

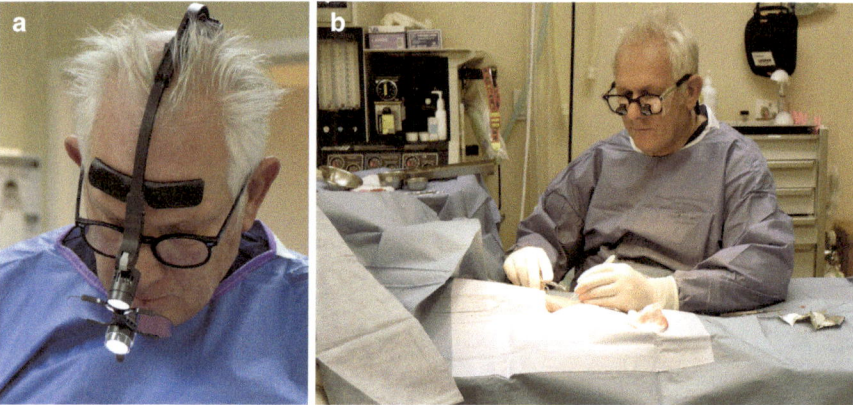

Fig. 3.1 Dr. Kim headlight with magnification and lead author operating under local anaesthetic on the LFJ Klaassen hand surgery table (est. 1988) with Designs for Vision surgical loupes, at a provincial minor surgery theatre suite.

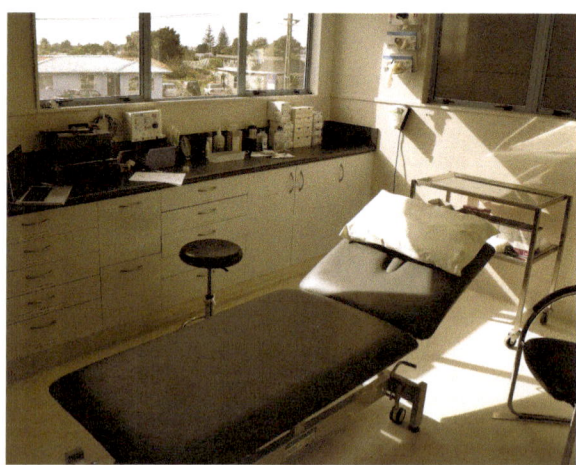

Fig. 3.2 Office minor surgery room

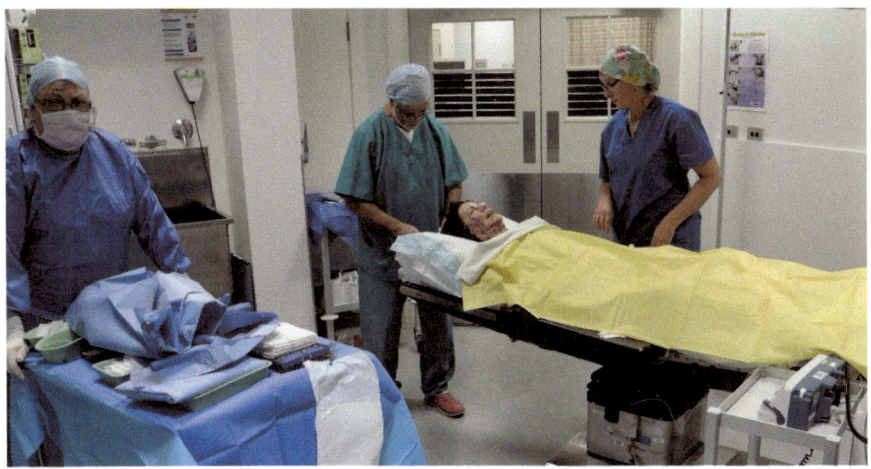

Fig. 3.3 Day surgery clinic operating theatre for GA and IV sedation cases

Standard Surgical Instruments

For most of my minor and moderate skin cancer cases, I use the same set of instruments. These are arranged on a Mayo mobile table and include no. #15 and no. #10 scalpel blades, Gillies skin hooks, Gillies tissue forceps, iris curved scissors for undermining and blunt dissection and Gillies needle holder for suture placement and suture cutting.

Depending on which region of the body is being operated on, the preparation solutions vary between sterile saline, Betadine and chlorhexidine (with and without alcohol).

Tip: Avoid splashing chlorhexidine in the eyes. It is very irritating to the conjunctiva. Consider preparing facial skin with saline or weak Betadine.

A bipolar diathermy unit is always available but is rarely used in my practice. This is due to the routine infiltration of local anaesthetic with adrenaline at least 10–15 min before commencing the first incision.

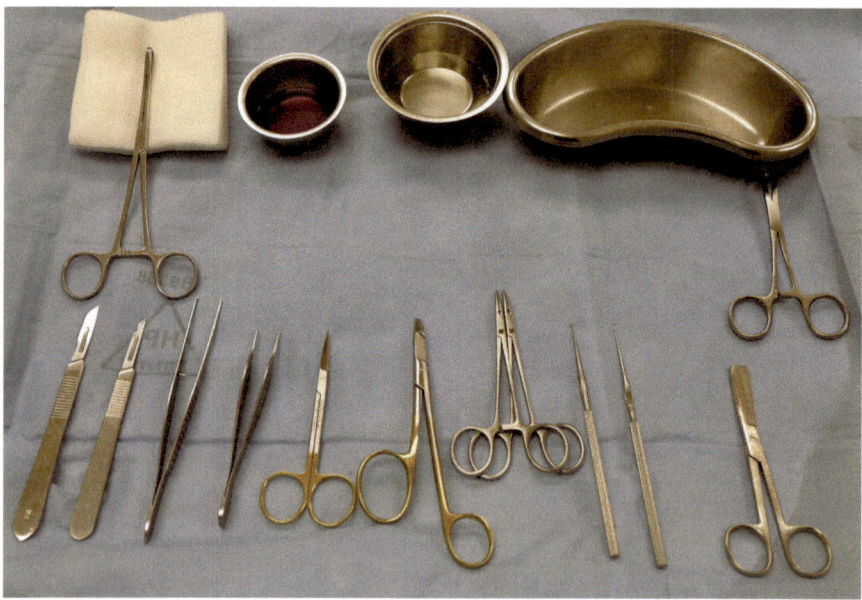

Fig. 3.4 Lead author's basic instrument set—sponge forceps, 10 × 10 cm gauze squares, chlorhexidine with alcohol, bowl of sterile saline, kidney dish for sharps, towel clip (optional), dressing scissors, Gillies skin hooks, mosquito forceps, Gillies needle holder, iris scissors, Adson tissue forceps, Gillies tissue forceps, #15 and #10 blades mounted on blade handles

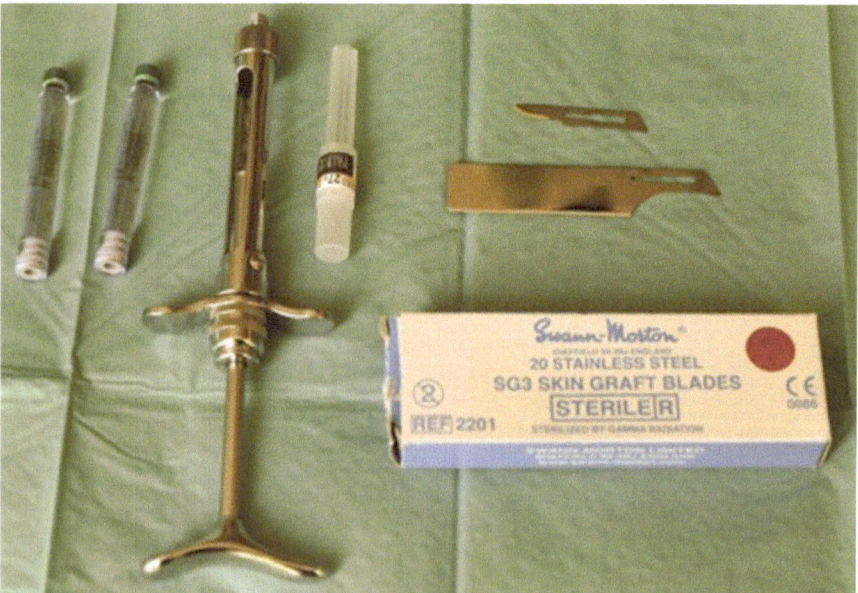

Fig. 3.5 Lead author's basic extras include—dental syringe with 27 or 30 G needles and prefilled cartridges for top up of local anaesthetic (if required). Swann-Morton surgical blades including the SG3 skin graft blade and the new Miltex silicone-coated #15 blade made by Integra. The precision cutting of the silicone-coated blades is a real advantage

Gentle Tissue Handling

This is a key principle always emphasized by Gillies [2]. The Gillies skin hooks are particularly useful for atraumatic handling of wound edges and local flaps.

Fig. 3.6 Gillies skin hooks advancing two keystone flaps for a shin defect

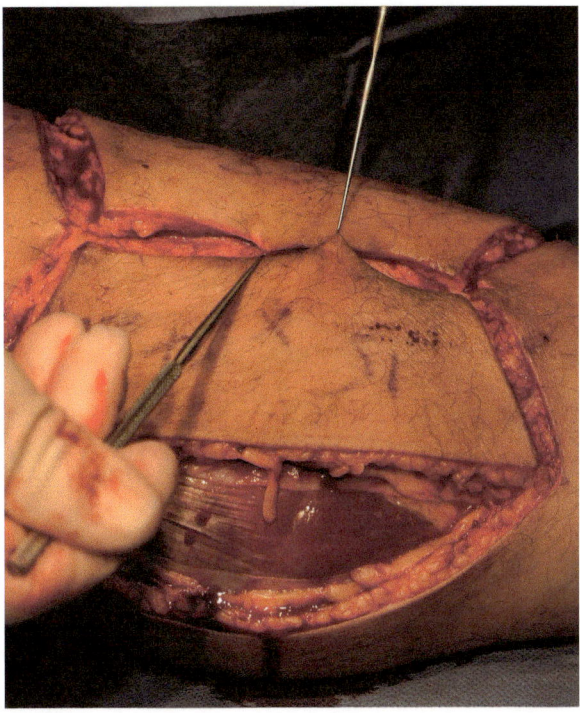

Suture Without Tension

This is especially important for the elderly with thin and atrophic skin. Leave some gaps if necessary, they will close by secondary intention healing.

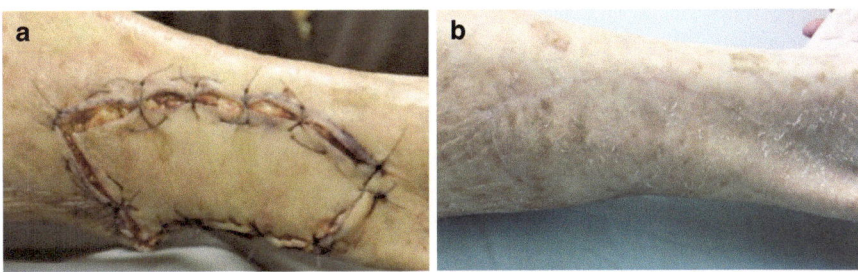

Fig. 3.7 Loose suturing of keystone local flap repair in a 94-year-old woman after wide excision of an ulcerated BCC (**a**) and 12 months post-operatively (**b**)

Photograph and Measure Everything for the Record, Especially Complications of Treatment

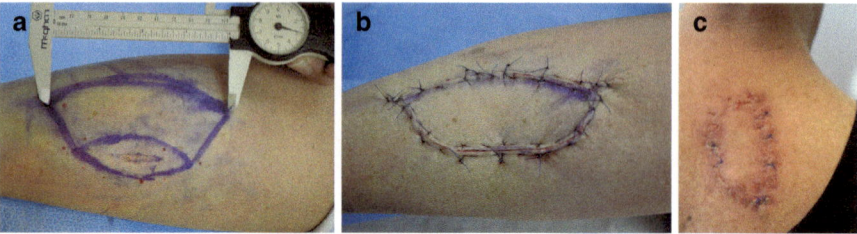

Fig. 3.8 Measure, record and photograph your surgery (**a**, **b**), especially complications like this inflamed keystone flap secondary to suture reaction (**c**)

Precise Surgical Dissection

This is important for mobilization of local flaps. I use sharp scalpel dissection combined with blunt scissor dissection.

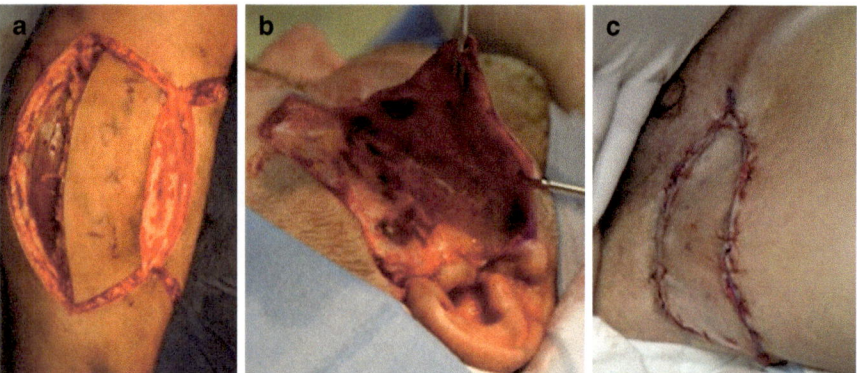

Fig. 3.9 Double pretibial keystone flaps (**a**), mini-facelift advancement flap (**b**) and large keystone perforator flap for paravaginal defect (**c**) all dissected with sharp precision

For keystone and other island perforator local flaps, it is important to avoid deep sutures. These will strangulate the perforator vessels and I never use them.

For most local flaps I recommend a change of dressing the following day, to remove blood-soaked wet dressings and replace with fresh dry dressings. This is especially important for patients taking anticoagulants (e.g. aspirin and warfarin).

Dressings vary between anatomical regions but for the local flaps to limbs (leg and forearm), I generally apply loose steristrips, absorbent gauze and then a padded crepe bandage. Elevation of the operated limb is essential for the first 48 hours.

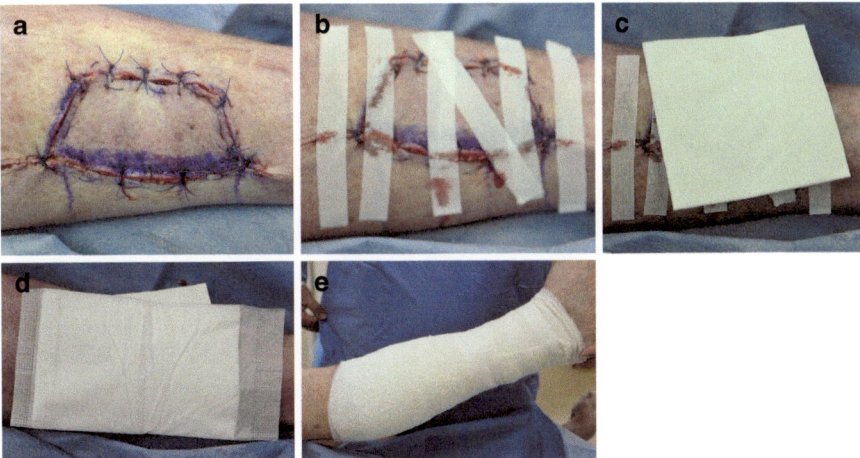

Fig. 3.10 Standard dressing for a keystone flap to a right shin defect (**a–e**). The dressings are routinely replaced 24 hours after surgery

For all patients, I recommend taping the healed scars with Micropore tape for at least 3 months after surgery.

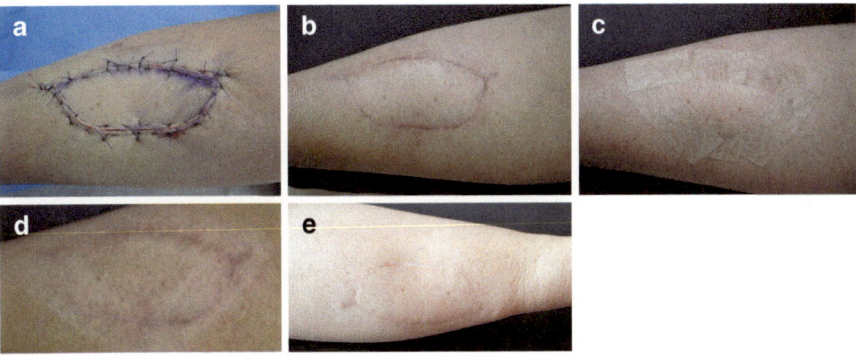

Fig. 3.11 (**a–e**) Scars of a keystone flap in a 62-year-old woman with melanoma right calf region immediately (**a**), after 1 month (**b**) and after taping with Micropore for 4 months (**c**, **d**), resulting in a satisfactory scar at 1 year post-operatively (**e**)

For early hypertrophic scars I use topical Cicacare (silicone gel adhesive pad).

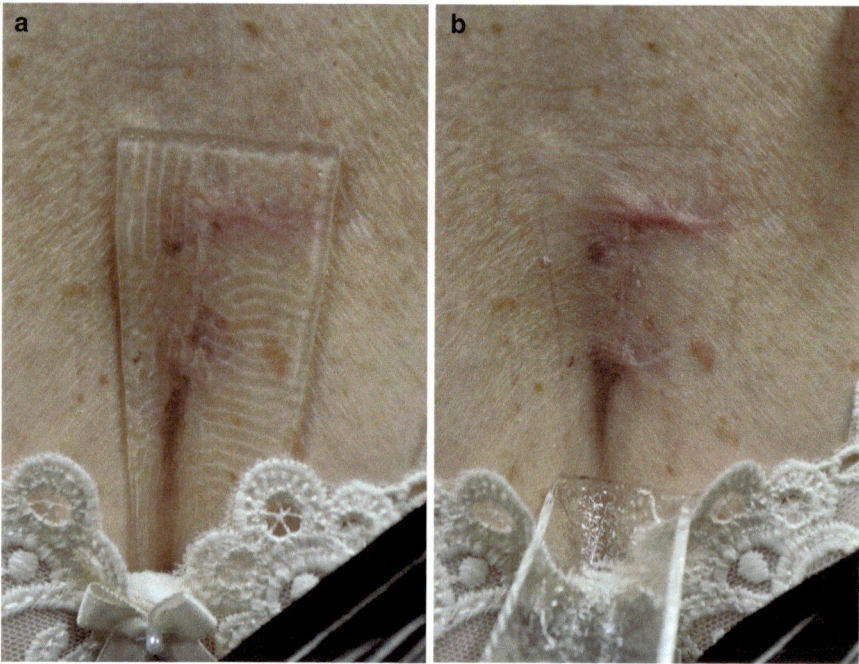

Fig. 3.12 (**a, b**) Cicacare silicone gel applied to hypertrophic presternal scar

For digital local flaps, finger tourniquets like the T-Ring or latex glove are helpful for identification of digital neurovascular structures.

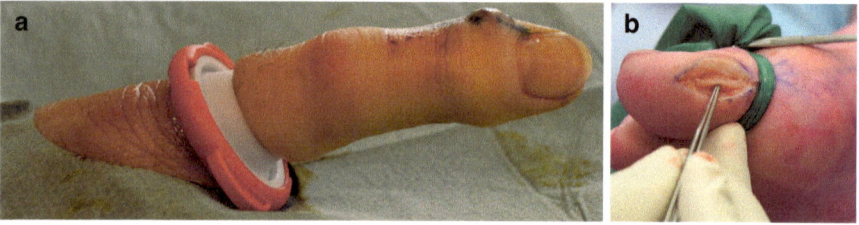

Fig. 3.13 (**a, b**) T-Ring and traditional surgical glove tourniquets to aid digital surgery

Designing a Local Flap to Avoid Tension in Hand Wound Defects

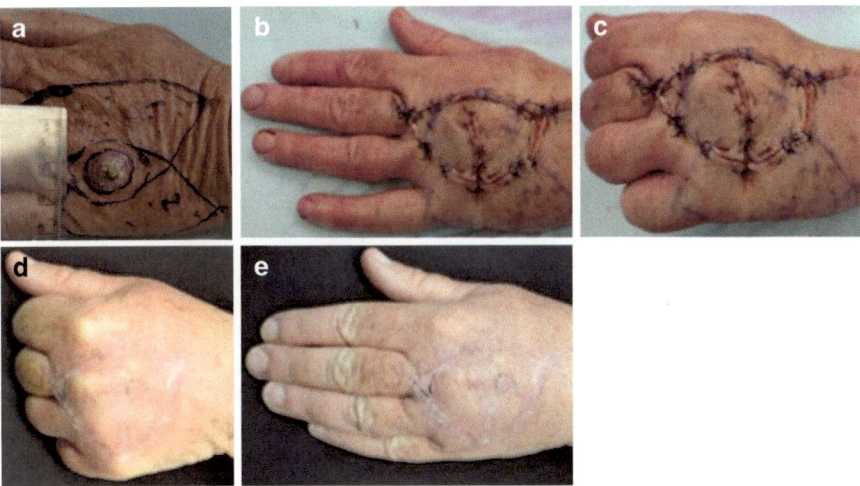

Fig. 3.14 A 58-year-old woman with well-differentiated SCC dorsum left hand (**a**), widely excised and repaired with a keystone local flap (Omega variant) to achieve tensionless closure (**b**, **c**) and preservation of hand function (**d**, **e**)

Managing Patients on Aspirin and Anticoagulants

If the patient is on regular aspirin or warfarin and has stable clotting tests (PT/INR), then I do not stop their medication, but warn them that oozing will be expected and a dressing change required the following day. Clopidogrel and other more powerful anticoagulants like rivaroxaban (a Factor Xa inhibitor) need to be stopped preoperatively at least a week in advance. Prescribing physicians (cardiologists and haematologists) are best consulted about this first.

References

1. Duke J, Keech B (2011) Anaesthesia secrets, 4th edn. Mosby Elsevier, Philadelphia
2. Gillies HD (1943) Technique of good suturing. St Barts Hosp. Med J 47:170–173

Part II

Traditional Local Flaps

Chapter 4: Elliptical Excision and Sliding Flap Repair
Chapter 5: Advancement flaps
Chapter 6: Rotation flaps
Chapter 7: Interpolation flaps
Chapter 8: Transposition flaps
Chapter 9: Triangular Flaps That Transpose, Advance and Interdigitate
Chapter 10: Hinge Flaps
Chapter 11: Recommended Traditional Local Flaps

Elliptical Excision and Sliding Flap Repair

4

Elliptical excision and sliding flap repair is the basis of all traditional local flap repairs and is one of the most common minor surgical procedures. Whilst it could be argued that such a procedure could be defined as a double advancement flap repair, it does not require any additional importation of skin to repair the wound or surgical defect.

The steps in this procedure are:

1. Assess the lesion and surrounding skin.
2. Outline the lesion.
3. Outline the proposed excision margin.
4. Determine and mark the relaxed skin tension lines (RSTLs).

    On the face, mark the facial creases with the patient sitting up or standing. On other parts of the body, mark natural creases or use Flint's circles.
5. Draw an ellipse to encompass the lesion and its excision margin.

    The long axis of the ellipse follows the relaxed skin tension lines (RSTLs) or facial creases when smiling or according to the Flint's circles, and perpendicular to the lines of maximum extensibility (LMxE).

    The ratio of length of the ellipse to the diameter of the lesion and excision margin should be no less than 4:1, to avoid dog-ears in the repair. The procedure is wasteful of normal skin amounting to about 75% of the total excision area.
6. Excise the ellipse of tumour-bearing skin.
7. Undermine the margins of the wound through subcutaneous tissue at the level of the base of the excision preserving the subdermal plexus and vascularity of the flaps. The amount of undermining is inversely proportional to the skin laxity. This undermining creates sliding or double advancement flaps.

    On the face, undermining should be kept just deep to the dermis, to avoid the underlying facial muscles and branches of the facial nerve. Undermining in other parts of the body can safely be done at the subdermal level for small excisions without compromising blood supply. For larger excisions, undermining of the scalp can safely be done in the plane between the galea and the pericranium, and in the trunk and limbs, the undermining plane should be either superficial or deep to the deep fascia.

© Springer International Publishing AG 2018
M.F. Klaassen et al., *Simply Local Flaps*,
https://doi.org/10.1007/978-3-319-59400-2_4

8. The wound margins are drawn together, initially with skin hooks to assess the amount of advancement obtained. The wound is then sutured to create a linear scar.

In a true ellipse, both sides of the wound are of equal length. Gentle handling of the skin edges and suturing by taking equal increments of skin and skin eversion should result in a good scar.

Mathematical Analysis

For a 1 cm diameter circular excision and an ellipse of 4 cm

    Area of circular excision of lesion = 0.8 sq. cm

    Area of ellipse = 3.14 sq. cm

    Area of normal skin removed = 2.34 sq. cm

    This is the equivalent of almost 75% of the total elliptical excision

---

Modifications of the Ellipse

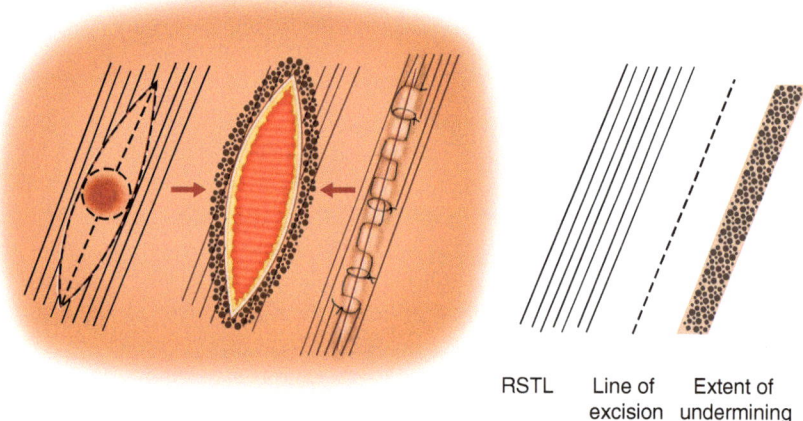

RSTL   Line of   Extent of
        excision undermining

Fig 4.1 Elliptical excision and double advancement flaps. The lesion (e.g. BCC) with excision margins and 4:1 ellipse in the RSTLs. Symmetrical undermining in subcutaneous plane and direct closure with double advancement (sliding) local flaps

In repairing an elliptical excision, symmetrical undermining is done on each side of the wound. In order to prevent distortion of significant landmarks, undermining on one side only is a good solution.

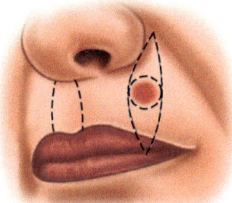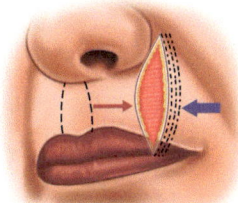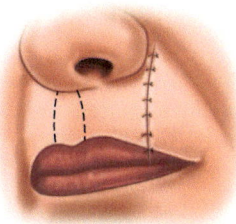

Fig. 4.2 Left upper lip tumour with excision margins drawn, a 4:1 elliptical excision in the RSTLs and closure after undermining the lateral wound edge for 4–5 mm to prevent distortion of the left alar base and Cupid's bow

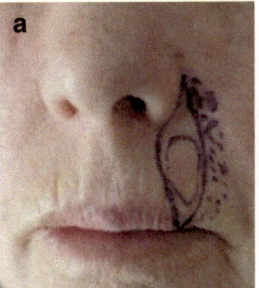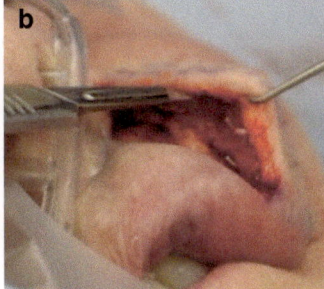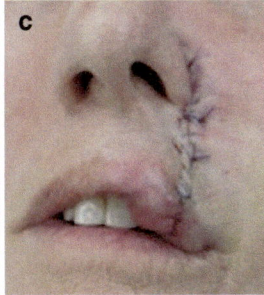

Fig. 4.3 Clinical example of a unilateral simple sliding flap from left medial cheek to left upper lip to prevent distortion of key anatomical landmark Cupid's bow in a 65-year-old woman (**a**). Unilateral undermining at the lateral edge (**b**) and final repair (**c**)

Fig. 4.4 Result 1 month following a unilateral sliding cheek flap to left upper lip

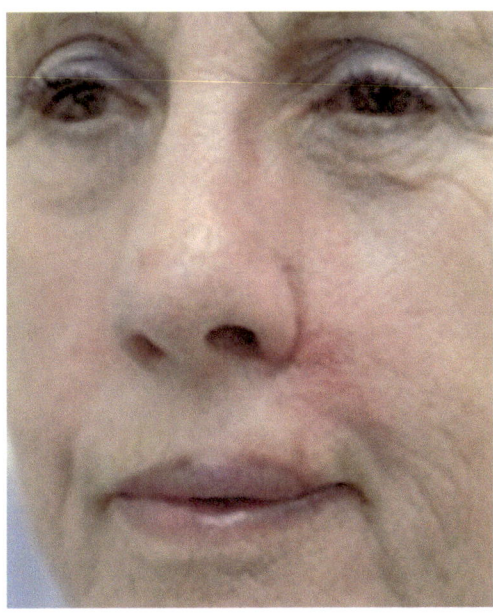

Crescentic Ellipse

The repair of a classical elliptical excision of a skin lesion invariably results in a straight line scar. In certain areas of the face, the ideal surgical scar should be curved, to fit in perfectly with the lines of facial expression or RSTLs. In order to achieve this, the ellipse can be modified in a crescentic fashion. When the lesion is excised in this manner, both sides of the ellipse are of equal length. Only the inner side of the ellipse is undermined before suturing.

Fig. 4.5 Crescentic ellipse design and scar

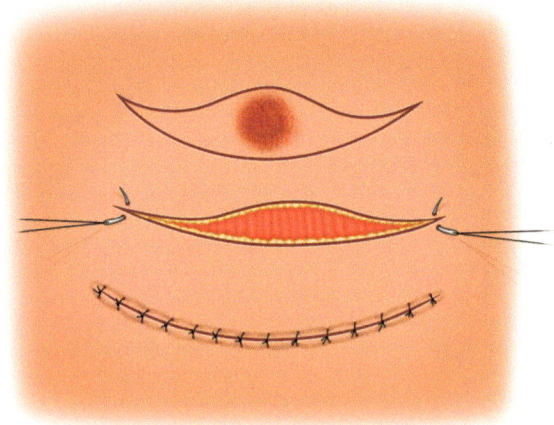

Asymmetrical Ellipse

In situations where there is an asymmetrical ellipse, with one side longer than the other, direct repair with sliding flaps may be difficult or even impossible, without producing a prominent dog-ear deformity. Where the difference in length of each side of the ellipse is not great, it is possible to carefully suture the wound by placing the sutures on the longer side, wider than those on the shorter side. In this way, the sides will equalise without producing a ruffle effect. Where the difference in length is greater, equalising the two sides can be achieved by reducing the length on one side or increasing it on the other. The longer side can be shortened by excising one or more triangles of skin from along its length. These are known as Symanowski's triangles [1].

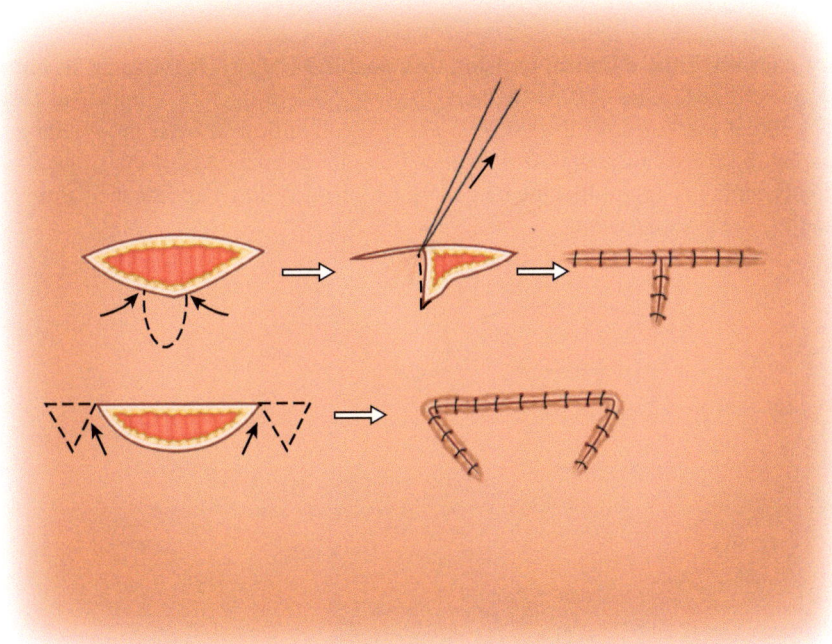

Fig. 4.6 Asymmetrical ellipse

Wedge Excision

This can be regarded as half an ellipse and applies to multilayered structures such as the lips, eyelids and ear [2].

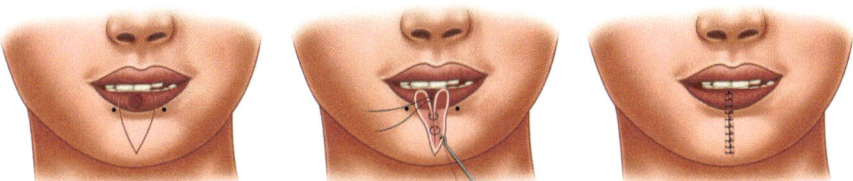

Fig. 4.7 Classic wedge resection/excision of SCC lower lip margin. The excision can be combined with an M-plasty and or vermillionectomy (lip shave) [3]

M-plasty [4, 5]

By converting the elliptical excision to a double M-plasty, the amount of normal skin sacrificed in the repair is reduced to about 50% of the total elliptical excision. The initial markings for the excision are as for an elliptical excision. A triangular flap with its apex of about 30° is planned on one or both ends of the surgical site. Undermining is done under the long margins. These sliding flaps are then advanced, and the wound is repaired.

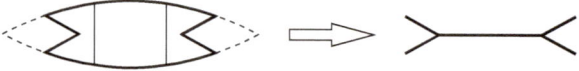

Fig. 4.8 Design of double M-plasty

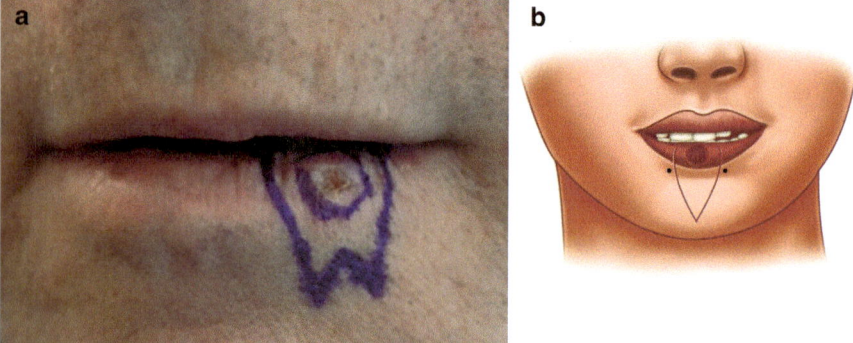

Fig. 4.9 Wedge excision planned for this SCC of the lower lip in a 55-year-old man and repair with M-plasty design (**a**). Classic tissue-wasting wedge excision, shown for comparison (**b**) [1]

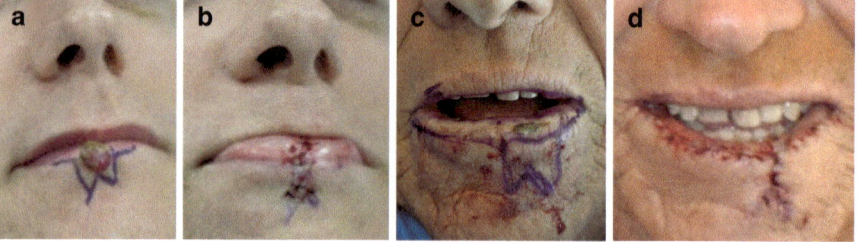

Fig. 4.10 Clinical examples of simple superficial M-plasty for pyogenic granuloma lower lip (**a**, **b**) and deep wedge excision combined with lip shave + mucosal advancement for SCC and dysplasia of the lower lip (**c**, **d**)

Crown Excision [6]

Fig. 4.11 Design and
scars produced by the
Robbins crown excision

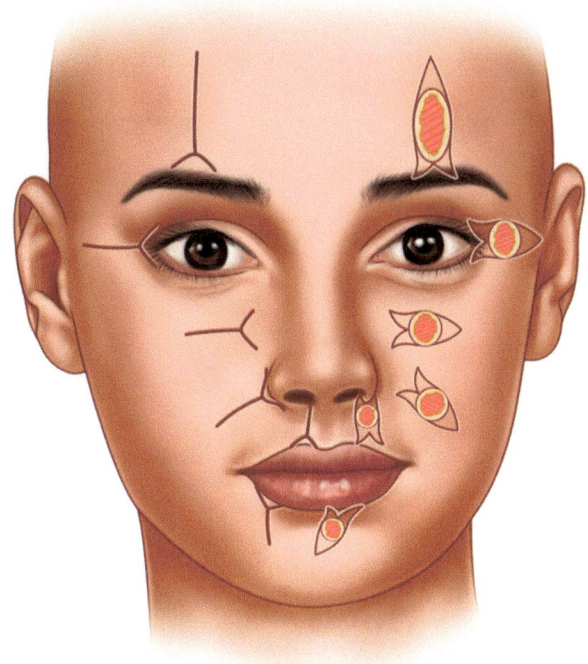

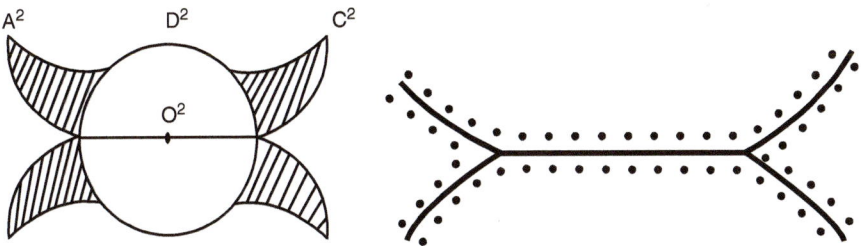

Fig. 4.12 Design of crown excision

This is another modification of an elliptical excision. It is particularly useful to
repair wounds close to important anatomical landmarks, where an elliptical excision
would distort these landmarks. Like the M-plasty it can be used as a double flap
repair on both ends of the excision, or as a single flap repair. Its planning allows for
skin edges of equal length ($A^2O^2C^2$ is equal to $A^2D^2C^2$) to be approximated.

Modifications of the Wedge Excision [4, 5]

The usual wedge or triangular excision involving free margins of structures such as the lips, eyelids or ear is wasteful of normal skin and can produce a notch at the free margin, if not repaired accurately in layers.

Clinical scenario: A basal cell carcinoma close to the right lower eyelid margin

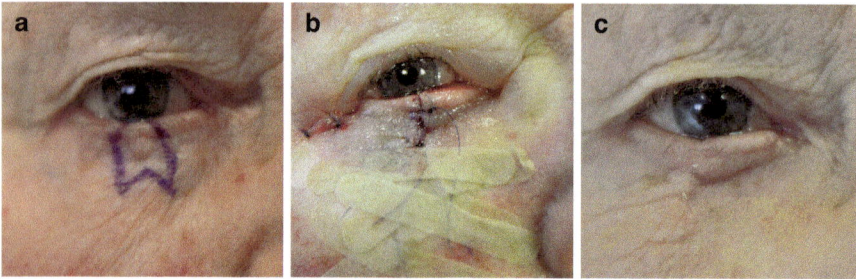

Fig. 4.13 Wedge excision of micronodular BCC right lower eyelid in a 70-year-old woman (**a**). Repair with M-plasty, double eyelid advancement flaps and three-layered Mustardé eyelid repair. Immediate (**b**) and 2-week post-operative result (**c**)

Surgical method: For this micronodular basal cell carcinoma near the right lower eyelid, a wide full thickness wedge excision was performed incorporating the M-plasty design to preserve tissue. Fine iris scissors are best for making the cuts either side of the cancer, and a lateral canthotomy is also performed, to achieve tensionless repair of the eyelid margins. A Mustardé three layer repair of the eyelid was performed with a continuous pull-out 5/0 Prolene to the tarsoconjunctival layer, orbicularis oculi approximation with 5/0 Vicryl and finally interrupted nylon to the outer layer [7].

The suture ends are left long and Steristripped down to avoid suture irritation of the cornea. The free margin of the eyelid is repaired carefully to avoid future notching.

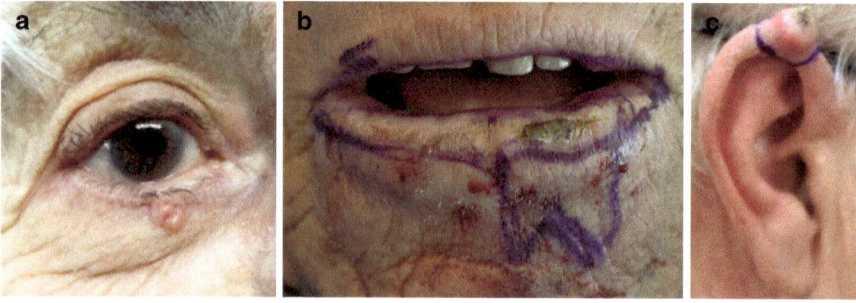

Fig. 4.14 Clinical examples of BCCs and SCCs at the free margins of eyelid (**a**), lower lip (**b**) and superior helix of the ear (**c**), where notching may result from a standard wedge resections

The method of rotation-advancement can be used to reduce the amount of normal tissue excised and reduce the possibility of a notch forming at the free margin (See Page 73, Fig. 6.18). More scarring is introduced, however, especially in the lower lip.

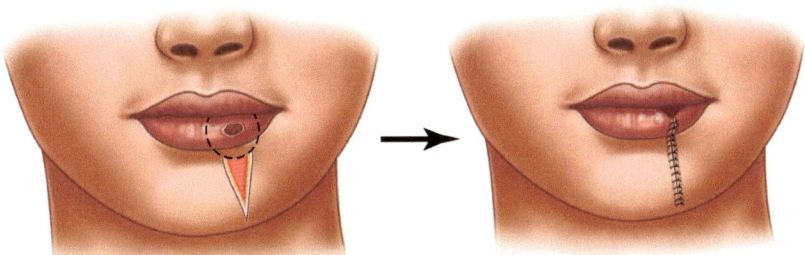

Fig. 4.15 Skin markings for wedge excision lower lip with notch result at free margin

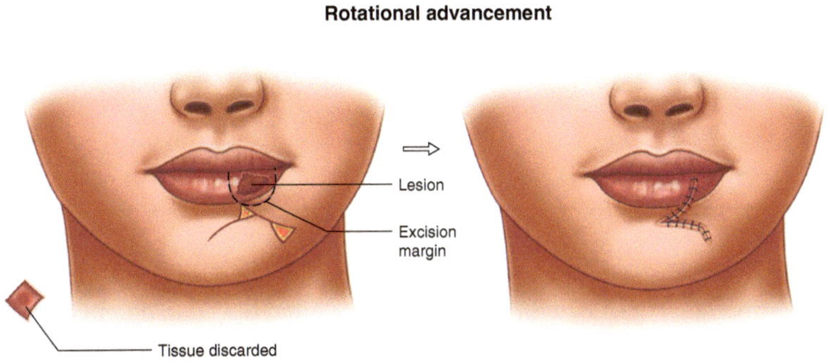

Rotational advancement

Lesion

Excision margin

Tissue discarded

Fig. 4.16 Rotation-advancement technique to reduce tissue wastage and risk of notching

Notes

When the surgical defect is created, the margins of the wound can be tested for skin laxity, gently pulling each with skin hooks. Should there be little or no laxity in the skin and the wound edges cannot be opposed, an alternative method of closure should be chosen.

In some cases there may be a temptation to oppose the skin edges under tension, to avoid a more complex repair. This can result in wound dehiscence or a hypertrophic scar.

In a true ellipse, both sides of the wound are of equal length. Gentle handling of the skin edges and suturing by taking equal increments of skin and skin edge eversion should result in a good scar.

In a wedge excision (or half an ellipse), the wastage of normal skin in the excision can be reduced by incorporating an M-plasty in the repair.

Where the lengths of the sides of the excision are unequal, it is possible to absorb the extra length by the *technique of halving* [4, 5]. The first suture is placed halfway between the ends of the wound. The next sutures are placed halfway between the central suture and the ends of the wound. Suturing is continued in this fashion until the wound has been completely sutured.

Discrepancies in wound length greater than those corrected by the halving technique require other methods to equalise the wound length.

Fig. 4.17 Technique of halving when suturing a wound

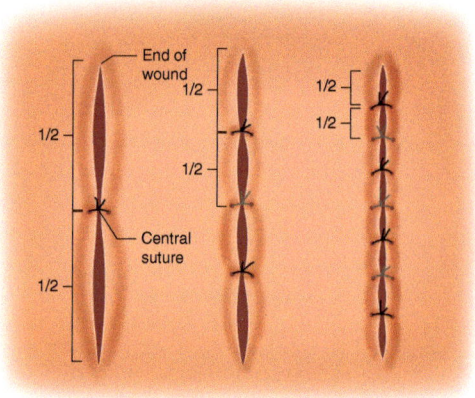

Dog-ears

These are standing cones of skin at each end of a sutured wound due to bunching of the skin. These can occur because the ellipse is too wide, too short, the wound sides are asymmetrical or the repair has not been done carefully.

The best time to correct a dog-ear is at the time of surgery [8]. The pucker in the skin is most unlikely to resolve with the passage of time as the surgical scar matures.

The simplest way of treating the dog-ear is to elevate the apex of a folded triangle of skin with a skin hook. Draw a line along the base on one side. An incision is then made along this line in line with the existing suture line. This creates an open triangular flap of skin that can be excised and the skin margins sutured.

This procedure will lengthen the final surgical scar.

If this measured approach to dog ear removal is not adopted, other methods can result in a much longer, uneven suture line. This approach is known as 'chasing the dog ear'.

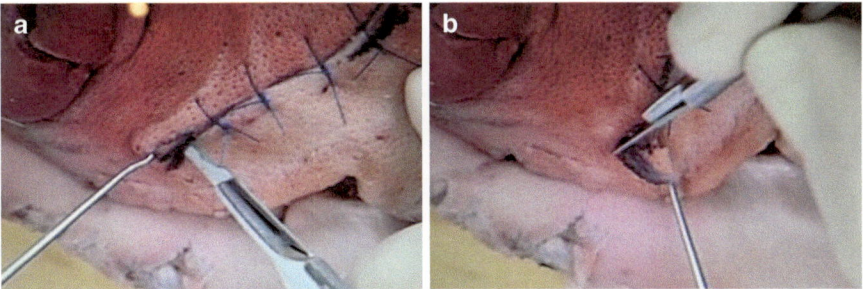

Fig. 4.18 Teaching demonstration of dog-ear excision on a porcine surgical model (**a, b**)

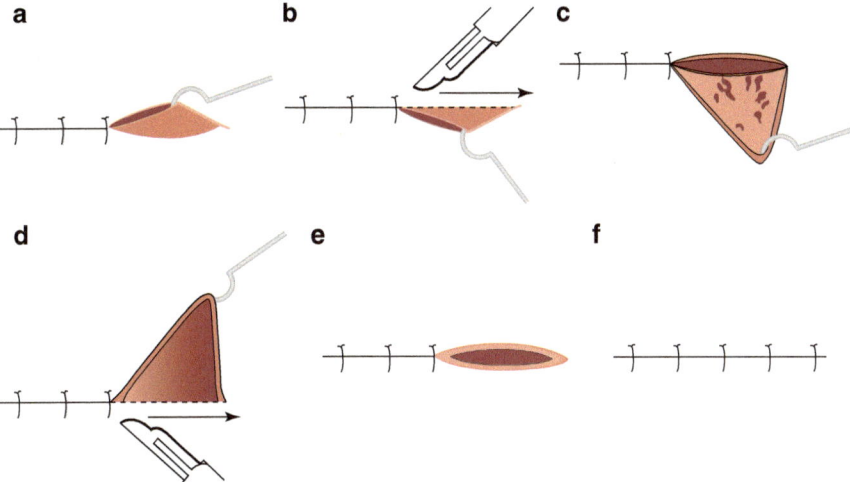

Fig. 4.19 Demonstration of one technique for dog-ear excision

Summary

The elliptical excision and repair is the basis of all surgical repairs. All the other local flap methods that follow are a natural progression or continuum, of this simple principle.

References

1. Symanowski J. von. Handbuch der Operativen Chirurgie. Viewegu Sohn, Braunschweig. 1870.
2. Johnson HA (1964) "V" Excision with less waste of normal skin. Plast Reconstr Surg 33(5):481–484
3. McGregor IA (1989) Fundamental techniques of plastic surgery and their surgical applications, 8th edn. Churchill Livingstone, Edinburgh
4. Brown, E. and Klaassen, M. (2011) Introduction to local flaps: a surgeon's handbook.

5. Klaassen, M., Brown, E. and Behan, F. C. (2016) Defining local flaps: clinical applications and methods
6. Robbins T (1976) The Crown excision of facial skin lesions. Plast Reconstr Surg 57:251–252
7. Mustardé JC (1991) Repair and reconstruction in the orbital region: practical guide, 3rd edn. Churchill Livingstone, Edinburgh
8. Jaibaji M, Morton JD, Green AR (2001) Dog ear: an overview of causes and treatments. Ann R Coll Surg Engl 83(2):136–138

Advancement Flaps

5

These flaps make use of the elasticity of the skin and soft tissues to repair the wound. The flap is elevated and moves forward in to the defect without any lateral movement.

Such flaps have a very long history and were described, with diagrams by Aulus Cornelius Celsus in his book *De Medicina libri octo* [1].

Now new substance is not produced at the place itself, but is drawn from the neighbourhood; and when the change is small this hardly robs any other part and may pass unnoticed, but when large, it cannot do so. Celsus c 25 BC—c 50 AD.

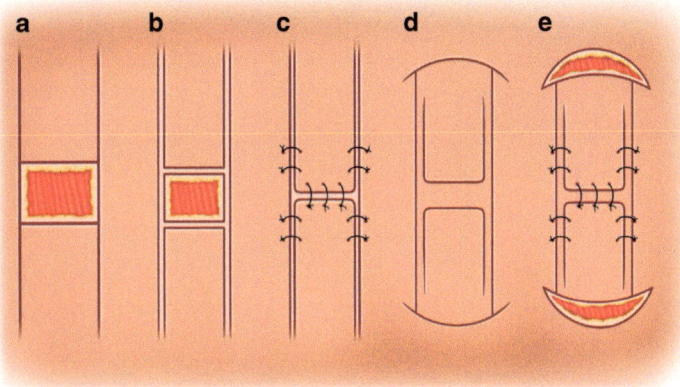

Fig. 5.1 Diagram of Celsus advancement flap

© Springer International Publishing AG 2018
M.F. Klaassen et al., *Simply Local Flaps*,
https://doi.org/10.1007/978-3-319-59400-2_5

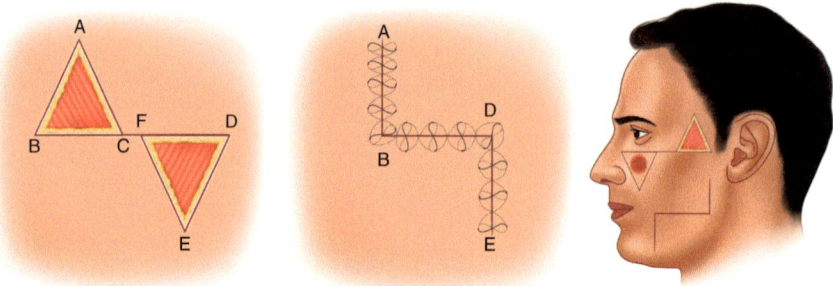

Fig. 5.2   Closure of defect by the method of lateral triangles after Burow [3]

A common technique in flap surgery is the excision of Burow's triangles [2, 3].

Early versions of the advancement flap left dog-ears at the base. Solutions to this problem by removing the dog-ears and further advancing the flap were made by Camille Bernard in 1852 and Karl Burow in 1855. Both surgeons proposed that a triangle of skin be excised from each side of the flap's base in order to facilitate its advancement and improve the final appearance of the repair. This technique is known as the Burow-Bernard technique, or in the English literature as Burow's triangles. Limberg [4] describes this technique as a supplementary plastic manoeuvre to close triangular and quadrangular defects. He noted that it was paradoxical that in order to close a defect, a nearby triangle of healthy skin, equal in size to the initial defect, was to be discarded.

Single Pedicle Advancement Flaps

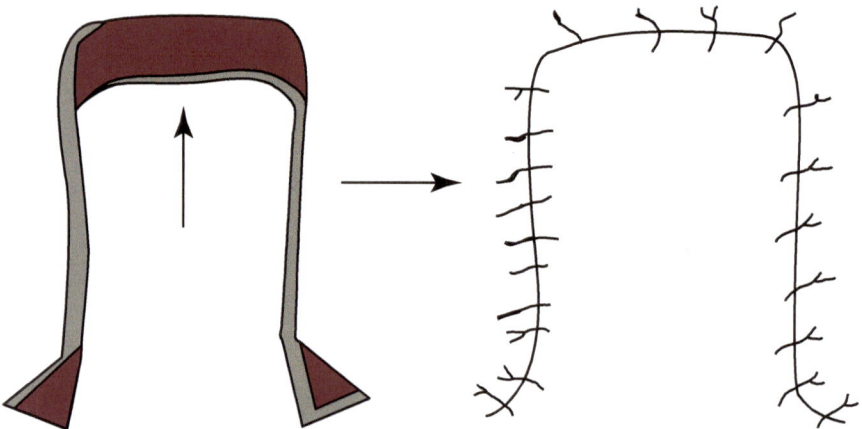

Fig. 5.3   Classical advancement flap with Burow's triangle excisions at base.

This flap is useful where there is laxity of the skin confirmed by the 'pinch test'. Burow's triangles have been drawn at the flap base to allow further advancement of the flap and eliminate dog-ears (Fig. 5.3). Theoretically the increase in the length of the advancement flap should be equal to the length of the lower side of the triangles.

The flap is created by making two parallel incisions extending from the rectangular surgical defect, ideally along the relaxed skin tension lines (RSTLs). The flap is elevated, and the margins of the wound and flap donor site are undermined. The flap is then advanced into the defect. This creates a discrepancy in length between the flap and the flap plus the length of the surgical wound.

Repair is by the principle of halves to spread the tension between the uneven sides of the wound. If dog-ears persist at the flap base, these can be excised by using Burow's triangles (extending laterally from the flap base) which would have the benefit of lengthening the shorter sides of the wound and preserving the maximum width of the flap base (where the blood supply enters) [5, 6].

In the past, much research was done on the ideal and safe 'length to breadth' dimensions of single pedicle advancement flaps. The tension on this flap produced by advancement decreases the blood flow to the flap. It is recommended that this flap be used in areas with an excellent blood supply such as the nose and scalp.

Where there is tension, but not significant enough to cause skin necrosis, atrophy can occur at the subcutaneous level to produce a depressed contour at the distal end of the flap.

Dorsal Nasal Flap

Classification: Advancement flap/single stage

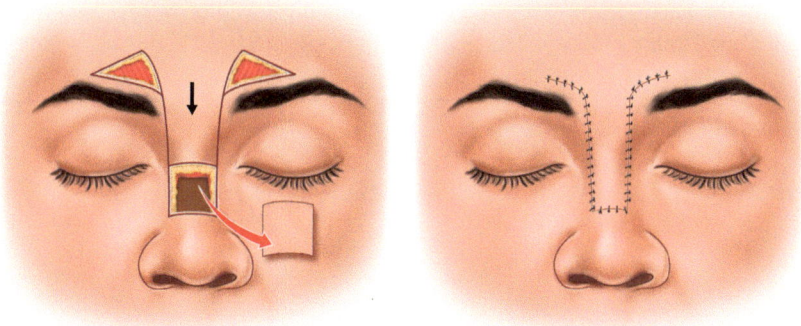

Fig. 5.4 The glabellar/dorsal nasal advancement flap with Burow's triangles [7]

Clinical case scenario: Basal cell carcinoma infiltrating supra tip of the nose in a 91-year-old man. Nasal skin laxity was an advantage in selecting this flap repair.

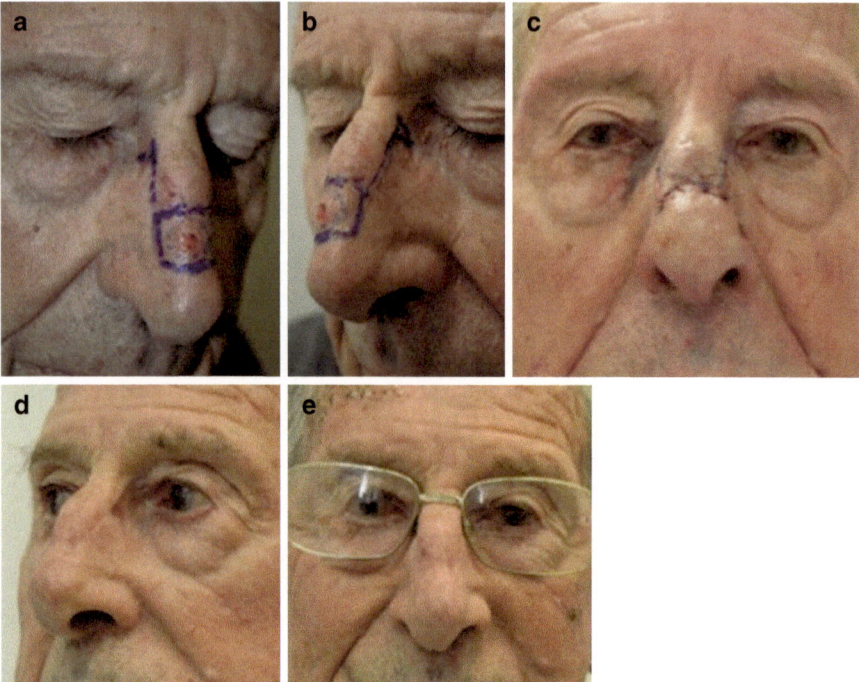

Fig. 5.5 Dorsal nasal advancement flap with associated Burow's triangles (**a, b**), early (**c**) and 2-year result (**d, e**)

Surgical method: The lesion was excised to create a rectangular-shaped defect incorporating the lower section of the dorsal nasal aesthetic unit. A dorsal nasal flap with Burow's triangles at its base was planned, raised and advanced in to the defect. Initially the nose looked foreshortened, but this improved with time, and the final result after 2 years is acceptable.

Mucosal Advancement Flap

Classification: Direct single pedicle advancement flap/one stage can be combined with a wedge resection of the lip.

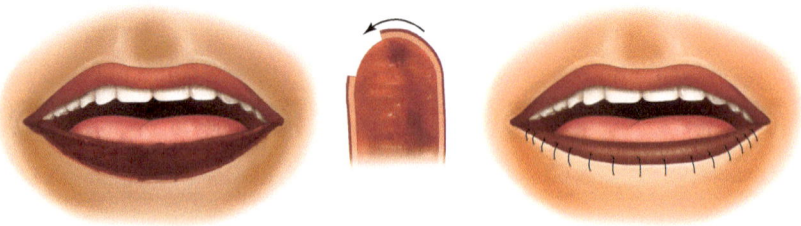

Fig. 5.6 Vermillionectomy (lip shave) with mucosal advancement [7]

Clinical case scenario: This 49-year-old male presented with a well-differentiated squamous cell carcinoma in the vermillion of the lower lip, associated with severe adjacent solar epithelial dysplasia.

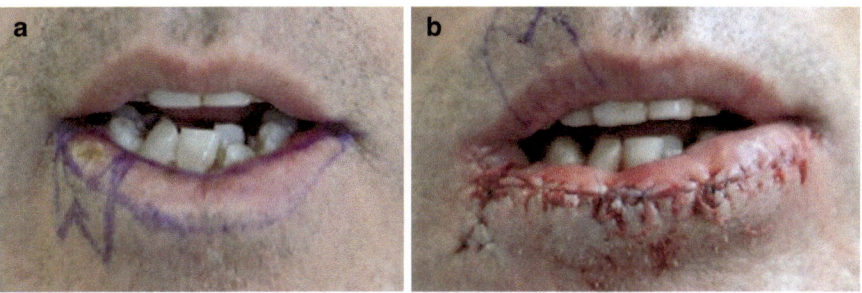

Fig. 5.7 Vermillionectomy (lip shave) of dysplastic lower lip combined with a wedge excision of SCC (**a**). An M-plasty is incorporated in the wedge excision. Immediate result (**b**)

Surgical method: The procedure was planned to include a full thickness wedge excision of the carcinoma and vermillionectomy in-continuity. The wedge excision was repaired directly, incorporating an M-plasty. A limited undermining of the inner lip mucosa was then done, and the mucosal flap advanced to cover the vermillion defect.

Notes

The combination of a tumour on the vermillion of the lower lip and extensive solar damage to the remainder of the lower lip vermillion is not uncommon. The excision includes the white roll of the lower lip plus the dry vermillion. Following this type of repair, the hair-bearing skin of the lower lip is in contact with the new vermillion.

Some authorities strongly advise that undermining of the mucosal advancement flap is unnecessary. The decision to undermine or not can be made at the time of surgery. We believe that several millimetres of undermining of the flap are helpful for its advancement and to avoid a tendency to post-operative entropion of the lower lip.

Double Advancement Flap

Biwinged Flap

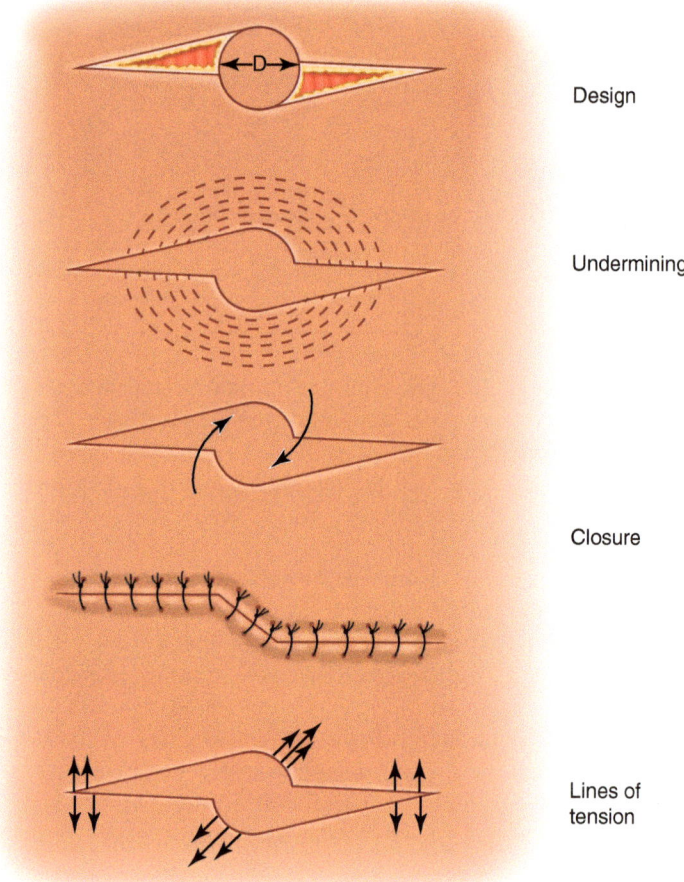

Design

Undermining

Closure

Lines of
tension

Fig. 5.8 Biwinged flap

Mathematical Analysis

For a 1 cm circular excision and the two wings equivalent to half an ellipse

Area of circular excision: 0.8 sq. cm

Area of square excision: 1 sq. cm

Area of one wing (half ellipse): 0.38 sq. cm

Area of both wings plus discrepancy between circular and square excision $0.38 + 0.38 + 0.2 = 0.96$ sq. cm

Percentage of normal skin excised in this repair is almost 55% of total excision

This compares with 75 % for an elliptical excision

Clinical case scenarios: Infiltrating basal cell carcinoma of the forehead

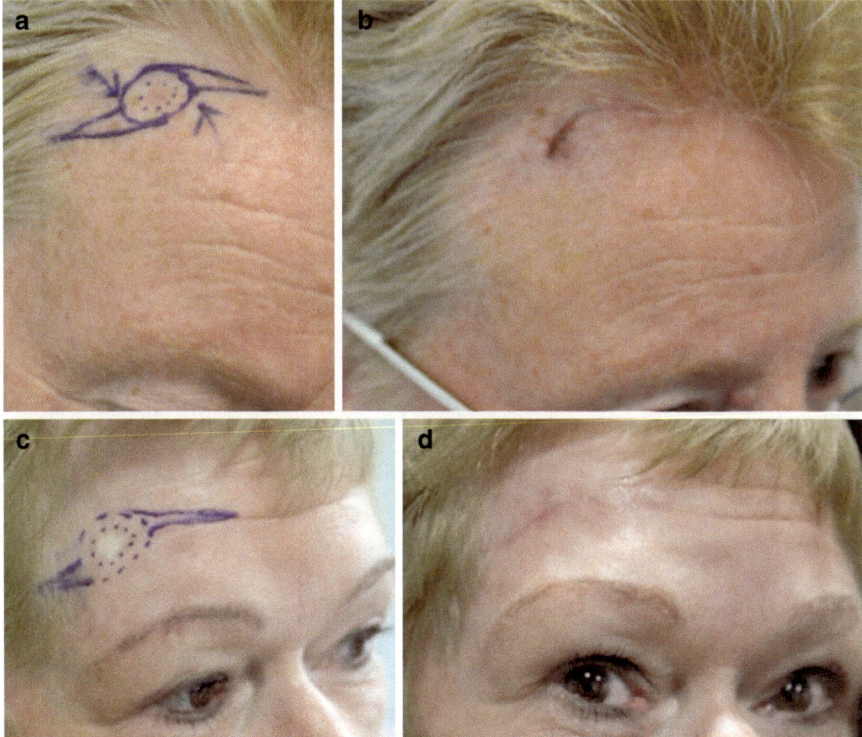

Fig. 5.9 Two clinical cases where biwinged excision techniques were used, to avoid distortion of the hairline and eyebrow. The upper is a nodulocystic BCC of the right upper forehead (**a, b**), and the lower is a sclerosing BCC of the right mid-forehead (**c, d**)

Notes

This technique is a variation of the elliptical excision. The wings of the ellipse can be placed according to the local landmarks. In this situation the wound is closed by advancing tissue on either side in to the defect and repairing the remaining wounds as sliding flaps. Differential suturing, taking a wider suture bite on the longer side, than the shorter side, is required to equalise the skin tension and give a linear scar. The final scar can be skewed on either side of the surgical excision, and this effect can be used to avoid distorting the hairline and eyebrow.

Perialar Crescentic Advancement Flaps

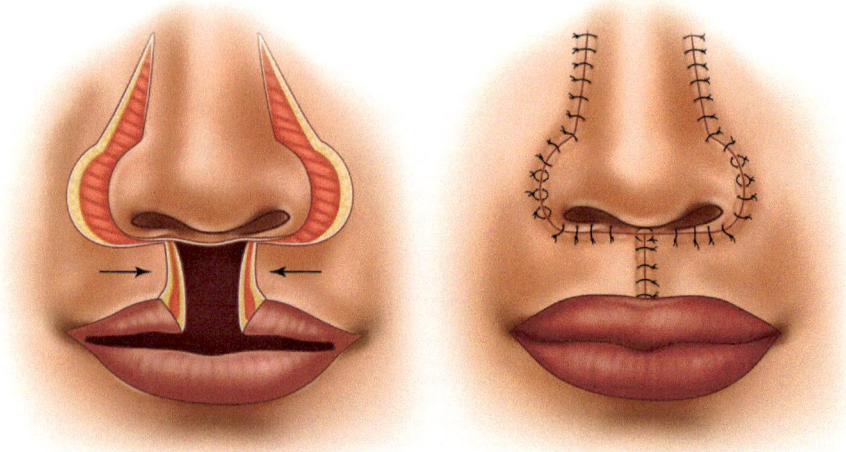

Fig. 5.10 Perialar crescentic excisions to facilitate repair of full and partial thickness defects of the upper lip [8]

Classification: Bilateral advancement flaps

   Clinical case scenario: Squamous cell carcinoma upper lip

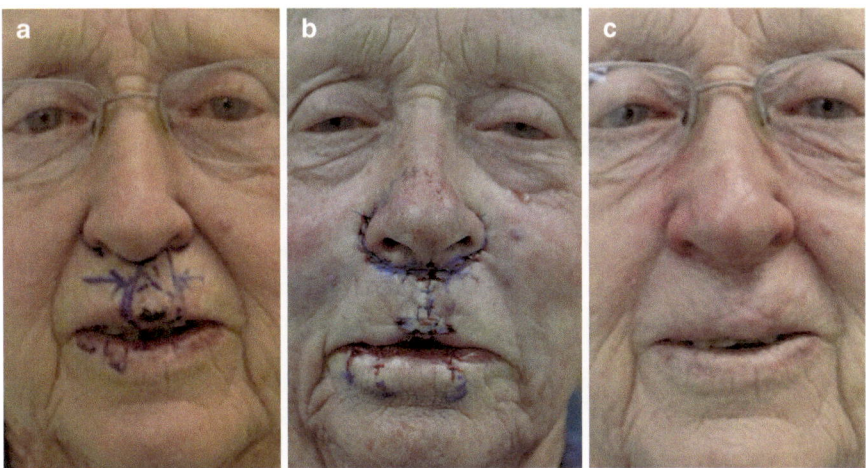

Fig. 5.11 SCC of central upper lip and philtral region, involving Cupid's bow (**a**), excised and repaired with bilateral perialar advancement flaps (**b**). Result at 6 months (**c**)

Surgical method: The squamous cell carcinoma was excised with a minimum 5 mm margin. The large central lip defect was then repaired using bilateral perialar crescentic advancement flaps. A small full thickness skin graft was used to recreate the Cupid's bow of the upper lip.

Notes

This is a good technique to repair larger full thickness defects in the central upper lip where direct closure is not possible. For more lateral lesions, the flap can be planned on one side only. Spare tissue for this flap is obtained from the nasolabial cheek fold. The alar base groove is retained. In the illustrated case, the pillars of the philtrum have been lost.

Double Advancement Flaps

H-plasty [5, 6]

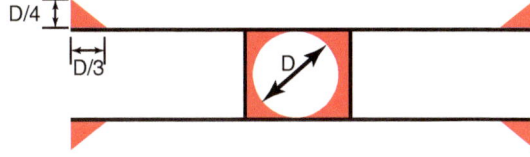

Fig. 5.12 H-plasty with Burow's triangles

This flap repair has two symmetrical rectangular advancement flaps, each covering half of the defect. The area of forehead above each eyebrow has more laxity than the upper forehead and, with the relaxed skin tension lines parallel with the frown lines, is an ideal location for this repair.

Classification: Double opposing direct advancement flaps with Burow's triangles

Clinical case scenario: A nodulocystic basal cell carcinoma right forehead

A direct sliding flap closure in a frown line would have elevated the eyebrow.

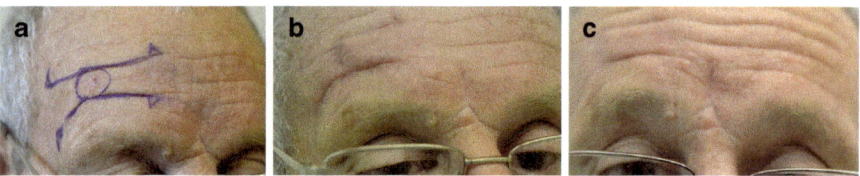

Fig. 5.13 H-plasty for BCC right forehead (**a**), 1 month (**b**) and 5 month results (**c**)

Surgical method: The surgical excision was planned to create a square defect. The H-plasty flaps, incorporating basal Burow's triangles were elevated in the direction of the horizontal frown lines. These flaps were then advanced to meet each other in the centre of the defect.

Notes

The forehead is an ideal place for this type of repair. The main flap scars are in the direction of the horizontal frown lines. If the flaps are too narrow, they can develop an unsightly trapdoor effect. This will tend to improve with the passage of time but will never completely disappear.

Flaps Involving V-Y Advancement [5, 6]

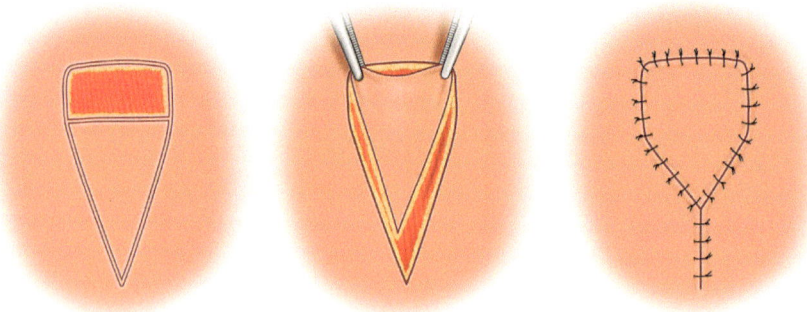

Fig. 5.14 V-Y advancement design. Gentle traction on the advancing flap should be done with skin hooks.

The principle is to plan a V incision with its linear base at the base of the rectangular surgical defect and advance the resulting triangular flap in straight advancement fashion towards the surgical defect.

The flap is based on the widest diameter of the surgical wound, and the amount of advancement required is the shortest length of the wound. In practice the excisional wound is converted to a rectangle. Where there is reasonable elasticity in the skin, the flap will be an isosceles triangle with an apical angle of about 30°.

Where there is poor skin elasticity, the triangular flap needs to be longer with a narrower angle at its apex to achieve the necessary advancement.

This flap is completely cut off from the subdermal vascular plexus, becoming an *island*. It receives its blood supply from the attachment of the flap to its subcutaneous tissues.

Undermining can be done on either side of the V flap to facilitate closure of the flap donor site as a Y.

There is an overall increase in skin tension in all directions, and the procedure does not give a great deal of advancement. The triangular flap is not stretched or pulled in to the recipient site but rather achieves its advancement by recoil or by being pushed forward. All the advancement occurs in the skin surrounding the V flap where it is sutured to create the stem of the Y.

This technique can be used to elongate structures like the columella, lower eyelid, lip and finger defects in the correction of Dupuytren's contracture. It can also be used to repair the philtrum or eliminate minor notches in the lip.

Nasalis Flap

Classification: V-Y advancement/single stage/island pedicle
Clinical case scenario: Small basal cell carcinoma lateral side of nose

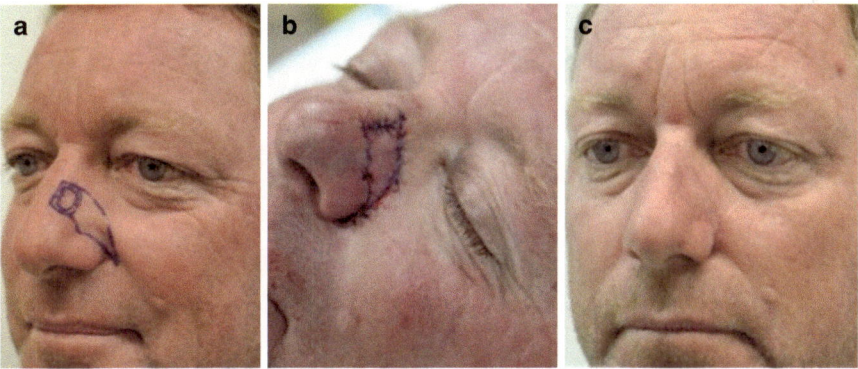

Fig. 5.15 V-Y advancement flap, lateral side of nose (**a, b**). Result at 3 months (**c**)

Surgical method: The BCC was excised with a 3mm margin up to the dorsal nasal subunit. A triangular flap was designed to follow the superior alar margin and crease. This flap was advanced in to the defect and the flap donor site repaired to create a final Y-shaped scar.

Upper Lip Case

Classification: V-Y advancement/island flap on subcutaneous pedicle

Clinical case scenario: Squamous cell carcinoma involving the Cupid's bow of the upper lip

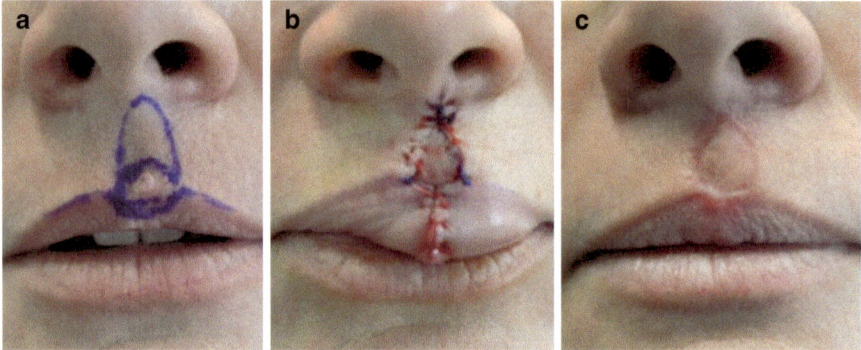

Fig. 5.16 V-Y flap in the philtrum of the upper lip for SCC in a 38-year-old woman (**a, b**). Early result 4 weeks after surgery (**c**)

Surgical method: The small squamous cell carcinoma close to the Cupid's bow was excised with a 5 mm margin. Reconstruction was performed with a V-Y advancement flap planned within the limits of the philtral aesthetic unit

Notes

This is a useful technique for repairing small skin defects or for structures that require some lengthening.

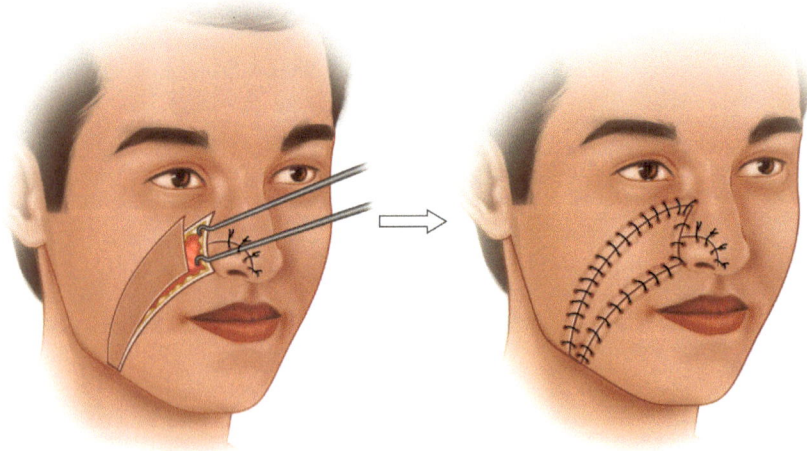

Fig. 5.17 Nasolabial subcutaneous pedicle flap

The V-Y advancement flap technique has been extended further for the repair of many facial defects.

Greater mobilisation can be obtained by converting the flap into an island on a subcutaneous pedicle. Careful dissection of the pedicle allows significant advancement, and the flap incisions are curved to follow the facial contours [9].

Sigmoid Oblique Advancement Flap [10]

Classification: Island pedicle advancement flap/single stage

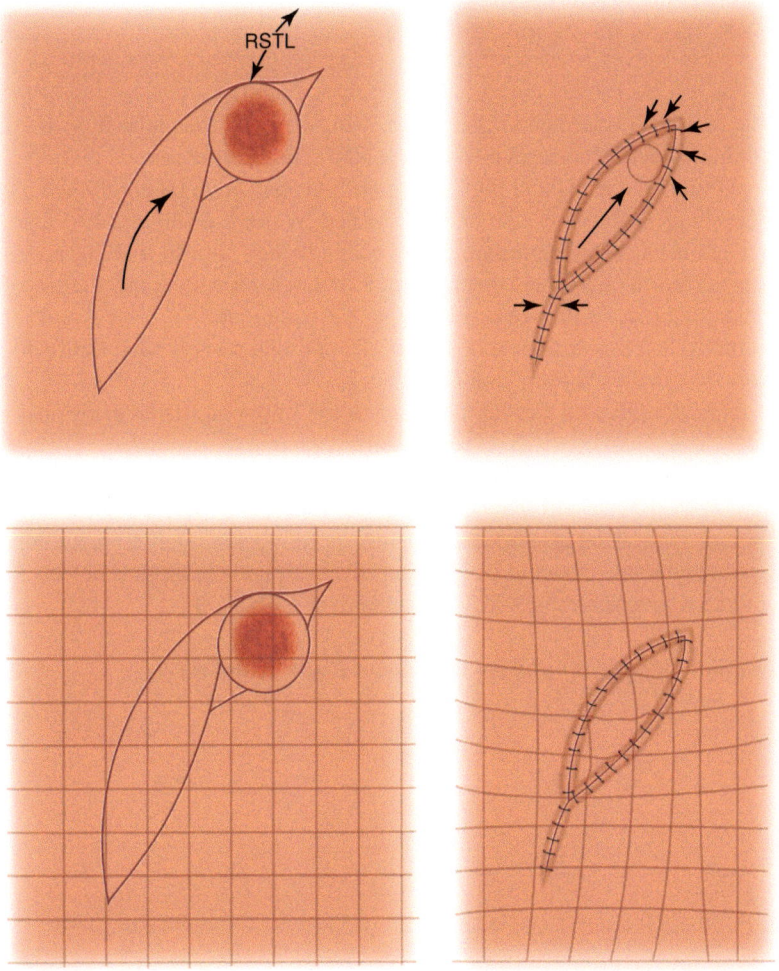

Fig. 5.18 Oblique island pedicle flap design and grid pattern foam block simulation from Ono's original article [10]

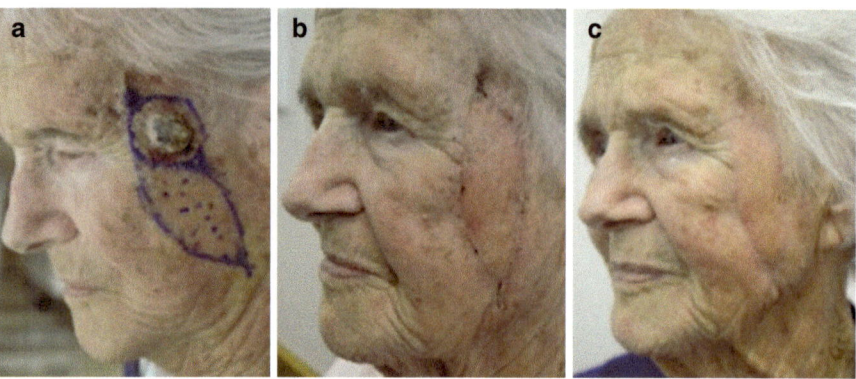

Fig. 5.19 Sigmoid advancement flap for an SCC lower left temple of a 91-year-old woman (**a**). Early result at 4 weeks (**b**) and 3 months (**c**)

The lesion is excised as a circle along with two small triangular flaps 1–2 mm in length in a direction corresponding to the RSTL or facial crease.

A sigmoid-shaped island flap having an S-shaped edge facing the defect and a spindle shape on the opposite side is planned. It has a width equal to that of the defect and is based on the proximal half of the defect, parallel with the crease line. The flap is raised on a subcutaneous pedicle and advanced obliquely in to the defect. The flap donor site is then repaired by the V-Y technique.

This flap has avoided some of the pitfalls of facial surgery such as trapdoor formation, depressed scars and dog-ears.

Placing the apex of the flap adjacent to the midpoint of the excisional defect reduces the amount of advancement required to repair the wound.

Surgical method: This large squamous cell carcinoma on the left temple was excised with a 5mm peripheral margin. The repair was planned according to the method of Ono. A large elliptical flap incorporating some loose preauricular skin was raised on a subcutaneous pedicle and advanced into the surgical defect. The flap donor site was repaired by V-Y advancement.

Smaller sigmoid oblique advancement flap for the face.

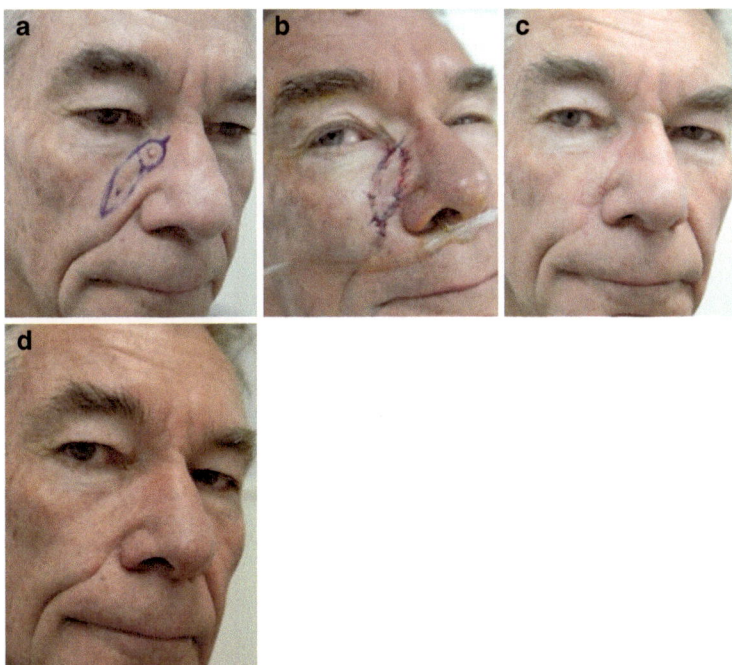

Fig. 5.20 Sigmoid oblique advancement flap for repair of a defect resulting from wide excision of nodulocystic BCC right nasojugal region in a 63-year-old man (**a**). The post-operative image shows the efficacy of the procedure where there is little skin laxity. Immediate (**b**), 1-month (**c**) and 2-year results (**d**). There is no post-operative ectropion of the lower eyelid

Double V-Y Flaps

Kite Flaps [11, 12]

In this procedure, two triangular flaps are raised on either side of the rectangular surgical defect. The flaps are incised down into the subcutaneous tissue, tapering outwards.

The two triangular flaps are then sutured together, and the defect was closed in V-Y fashion. The tension of the closure lies in the wound on either side, and the flap has minimal tension. Double sigmoid oblique advancement flaps of Ono can be used in a similar fashion.

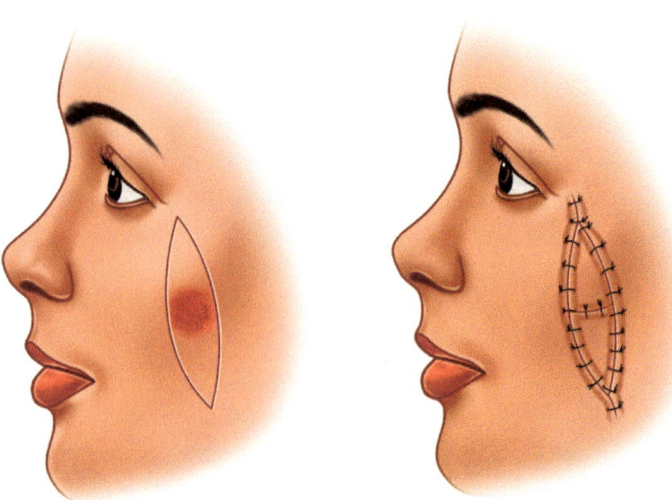

Fig. 5.21 Double kite flaps

V-Y Technique for Closing Surgical Wounds

A number of flap repairs leave a triangular donor defect. These can be closed directly by a V-Y plasty. These include the Hatchet flap, keystone perforator island flap and others.

The V-Y Technique for Releasing Scar Contractures [5, 13]

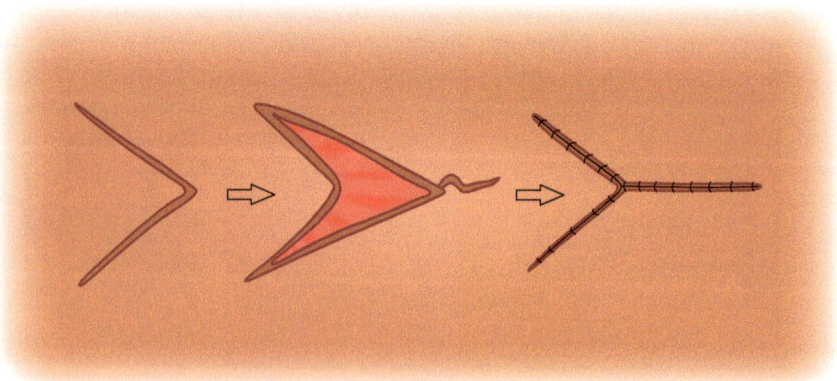

Fig. 5.22 V-Y design for scar release

V-Y advancement as an adjunct to Z-plasty.
In severe Dupuytren's disease, considerable improvement can be obtained to contractures with Z-plasties. In some situations the transposed triangular flap will not reach the apex of the wound, and a V-Y repair is necessary.

Y-V Advancement [5]

This is the opposite to the V-Y advancement. The main purpose is to gain width at the expense of length. The wider the angle of the triangular flap, the greater the increase in width. However, this is associated with increased difficulty in advancing the flap.

This type of repair can be used to correct epicanthal folds, digital contractures in Dupuytren's disease and some burn scar contractures.

A Y-shaped incision is made forming a triangular flap. This is then advanced into the stem of the Y, and the wound is then sutured as a V. The lateral skin borders of the triangular flaps are shorter than the total length of the Y, and there will be redundant tissue present after the advancement. To prevent this, Burow's triangles are excised on each side.

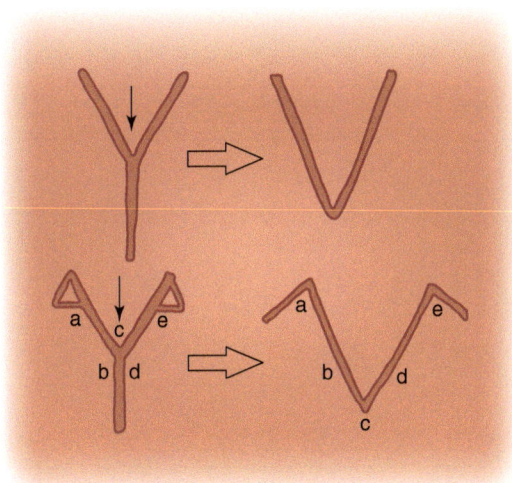

Burow's triangles excise redundant tissue after advancement

Fig. 5.23 Y-V advancement concept design

Multiple Y-V Advancement Flaps [5]

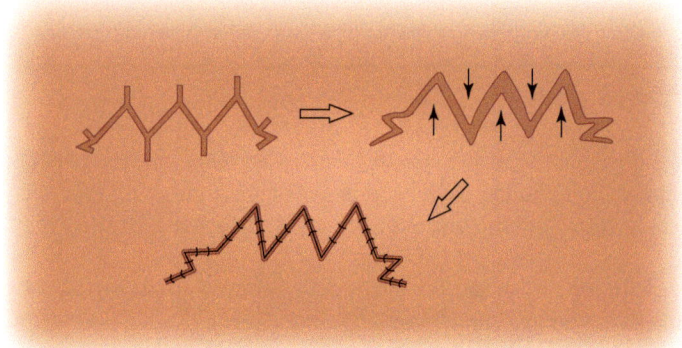

Fig. 5.24 Multiple Y-V design for scar release

The redundant tissue on each side of the advancement was excised as Burow's triangles, and these wounds were repaired with Z-plasties.

This technique can be used to improve broad scar contractures, especially lateral trunk burn scars, where Z-plasties would not be indicated.

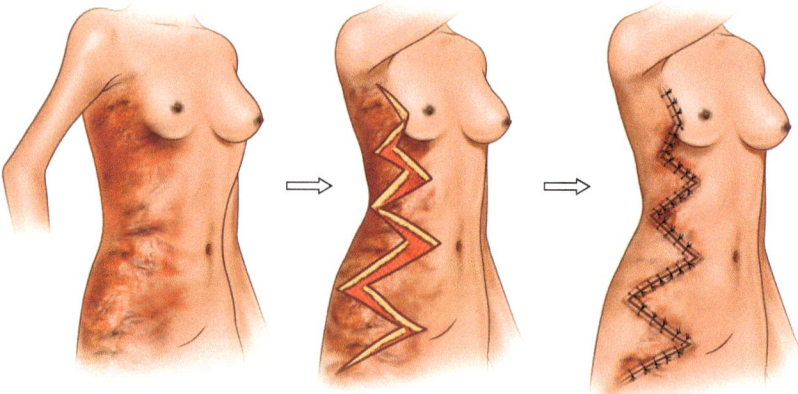

Fig. 5.25 Multiple Y-V advancement flaps for lateral chest burn scar contractures

Bipedicle Advancement Flap [5]

This strap-shaped flap is simple to plan and execute, having theoretically excellent viability due to its two pedicles. It can be regarded as two separate flaps joined at the centre EF.

The pivot points are A and C. When advanced, the midpoint of the flap F could fall short of the midpoint of the defect G unless under tension.

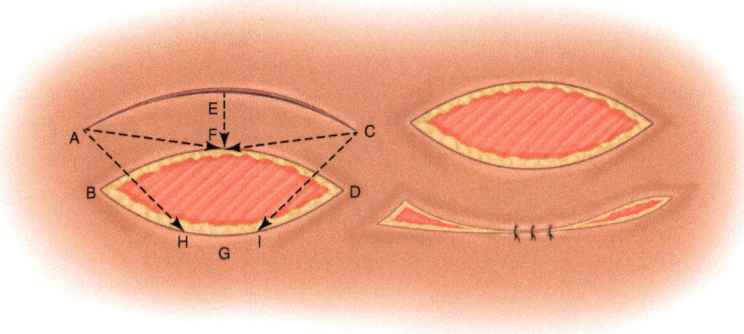

Fig. 5.26 Bipedicled skin flap design

Note

Many years ago, the bipedicle advancement flap was frequently advocated for repair of trochanteric pressure areas and exposed bone over the tibia following trauma. Unless the defect was very narrow or the skin was very lax, this type of repair was seldom successful. The amount of tension required to advance the flap into the defect resulted in wound dehiscence or vascular insufficiency. Safer flaps are now available for correcting these defects.

This flap is useful in lower eyelid repair, with the flap raised in the very extensible skin and underlying orbicularis muscle in the upper eyelid [14]. As the flap has to pass over the eye to the lower lid, it is best classified as an interpolation flap.

References

1. Celsus A C (47 AD) De Medicina (with English translation from Latin by W G Spencer Volume 111 MCMLXI London: William Heinemann. Cambridge: Harvard University Press.
2. Santoni-Rugui P, Sykes P (2007) A history of plastic surgery. Springer, Berlin
3. Goldwyn RM (1984) Carl August Burow. Plast Reconstr Surg 73(4):687–690
4. Limberg AA. The planning of local plastic operations on the body surface-theory and practice. (Translated by S. A. Wolfe, 1984); 1946. Lexignton: The Collamore Press.

5. Brown E. and Klaassen M. (2011), Introduction to local flaps: a surgeons handbook.
6. Klaassen M., Brown E. and Behan F.C. (2016), Defining Local Flaps Clinical Applications and Methods.
7. McGregor IA (1989) Fundamental Techniques of Plastic Surgery and their surgical applications, 8th edn. Churchill Livingstone
8. McCarthy J. G. (1990), Plastic Surgery. Volume 3, W B Saunders Company
9. Herbert DC, De Geus JJ (1975) Nasolabial subcutaneous pedicle flaps. Br J Plast Surg 28:90
10. Ono I, Gunji H, Sato M, Kaneko F (1993) Use of the oblique island flap in excision of small facial tumours. Plast Reconstr Surg 91(7):1245–1251
11. Emmett AJJ, O'Rourke MGE (1991) Malignant Skin Tumours. Churchill Livingstone, Second Edition
12. Strauch B, Vasconez LO, Herman CK, Lee BT (2015) Grabb's Encyclopedia of Flaps, 4th edn. Lippincott Williams & Wilkins
13. Andrades PR, Calderon W, Leniz B, Danilla S, Benitez S (2005) Geometric analysis of the V-Y advancement flap and its clinical applications. Plast Reconstr Surg 115(6):1582–1590
14. Manchester WM (1951) A simple method for repair of full thickness defects of the lower eyelid with special reference to the treatment of neoplasms. Br J Plast Surg 3:252–263

Rotation Flaps

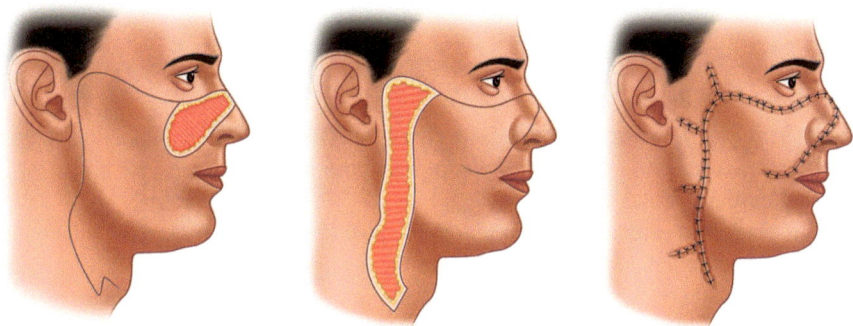

6

Fig. 6.1 Rotationplasty. Cover of a partial defect of the lateral nose and adjacent cheek based on original diagram of Esser, 1918 [1]

A rotation flap is a semicircular flap that moves on a pivot point. It is planned in such a way as to include any excess tissues within its dimensions and to incorporate a triangular surgical defect as a sector of the semicircle. This flap involves a pivot point, an arc of rotation and the diameter of the arc as its line of greatest tension. Its large base, at least three times longer than the length of the defect, ensures a good blood supply [2]. Planning of a classical rotation flap in theory appears deceptively easy, based on the similar diagrams repeated in the plastic surgery literature.

© Springer International Publishing AG 2018
M.F. Klaassen et al., *Simply Local Flaps*,
https://doi.org/10.1007/978-3-319-59400-2_6

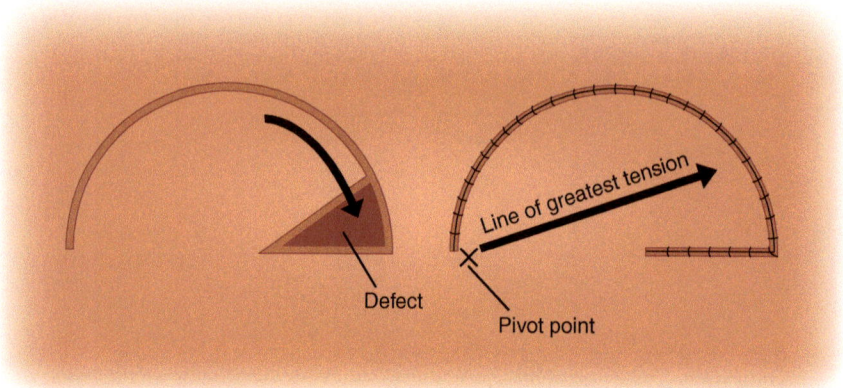

Fig. 6.2 Classical rotation flap

The initial defect is converted into a triangle. The flap is then planned so that one side of the triangle is adjacent to the flap, and the base of the triangle is part of the circumference of the flap.

In practice it is recommended that the flap be slightly larger than the plan so that when rotated, the flap will sit readily into the triangular defect under little or no tension. The distance from the pivot point to the farthest end of the flap should be equal to the distance from pivot point to farthest point of the defect.

When the flap has been raised and rotated, there is a difference in tension on the two sides of the wound due to their different lengths. Ideally this difference in tension is distributed evenly all along the suture line by the suturing technique of halving. The larger the arc of the circle, the longer is the line along which the tension difference can be distributed and the smaller the tension difference at any one point [3].

A small increase in mobility of the flap can be obtained by shifting the pivot point with a back-cut or by excising a small Burow's triangle. The back-cut shifts the pivot point towards the defect but has the effect of reducing the blood supply to the flap.

For large surgical defects, it may not be possible to completely close the flap wound, and a skin graft repair may be necessary.

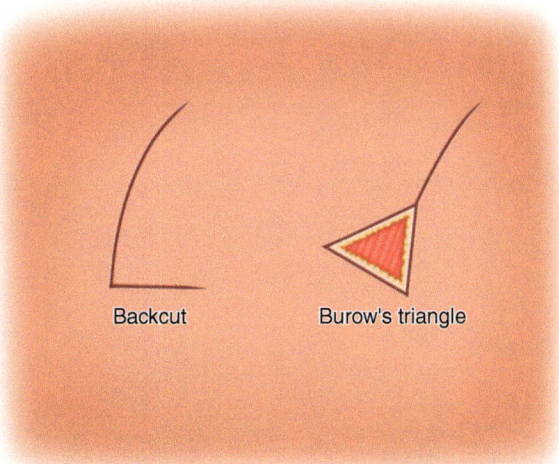

Backcut   Burow's triangle

Fig. 6.3 Moving the pivot point

Rotation Flap to Scalp

Classification: Rotation flap/single stage/flaps that move about a pivot point

Clinical case scenario: Recurrent basal cell carcinoma arising in an old scar on the scalp

Surgical method: The basal cell carcinoma and scar were excised with a 5 mm margin, and a scalp rotation flap was planned, raised and rotated in to the surgical defect.

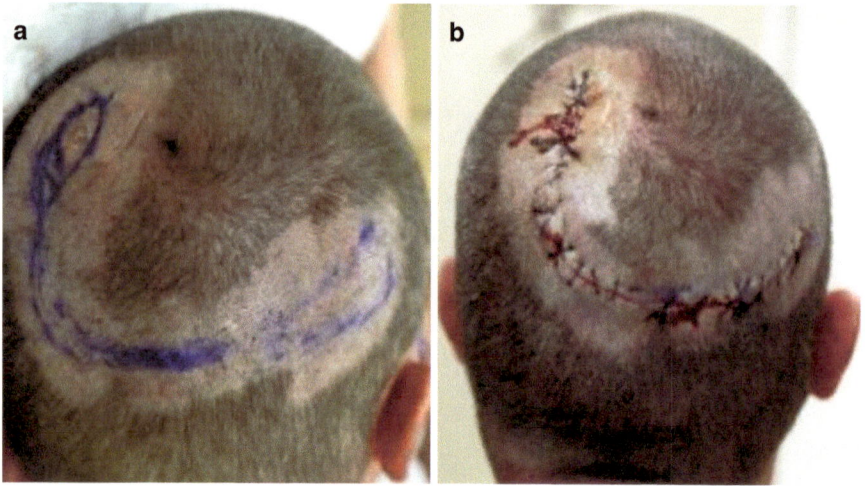

Fig. 6.4 Posterior scalp rotation flap for recurrent BCC in an old scar (**a, b**)

Rotation Flap Requiring a Skin Graft to Repair Flap Donor Site

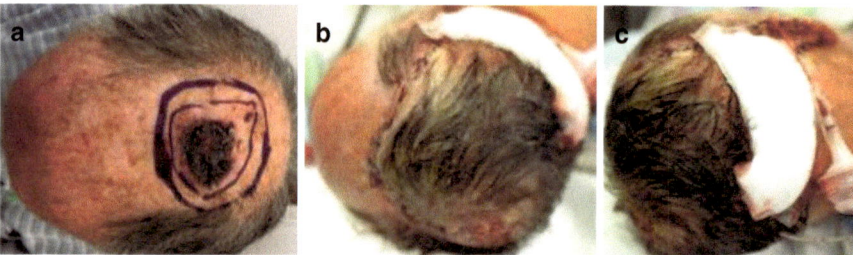

Fig. 6.5 Large SCC of vertex scalp in a 73-year-old man (**a**), widely excised down to calvarium and repaired with a large posterior scalp rotation flap based on the left occipital vessels (**b**). Split skin graft was used to repair the secondary defect (**c**)

Rotation Flap in the Temporal Area

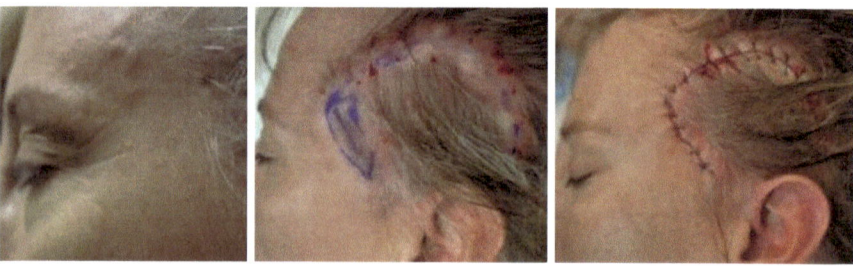

Fig. 6.6 A malignant melanoma in-situ in the left temple of a 45-year-old woman (**a**) was widely excised and repaired with a scalp rotation flap (**b, c**)

Notes

A rotation flap is a fairly large operation to correct a small defect. However, pedicled on a wide base, it is a safe way to redistribute 'like tissues'. For the scalp it replaces the defect with hair-bearing skin and covers exposed bone. Where there is insufficient elasticity in the flap to distribute the tension in a repair, a skin graft is required to repair the flap donor site.

The pivot point can be moved by a back-cut to increase the amount of rotation. The three-dimensional shape of the scalp makes precise planning and the avoidance of a skin graft difficult.

Rotation Flap for Buttock Defects

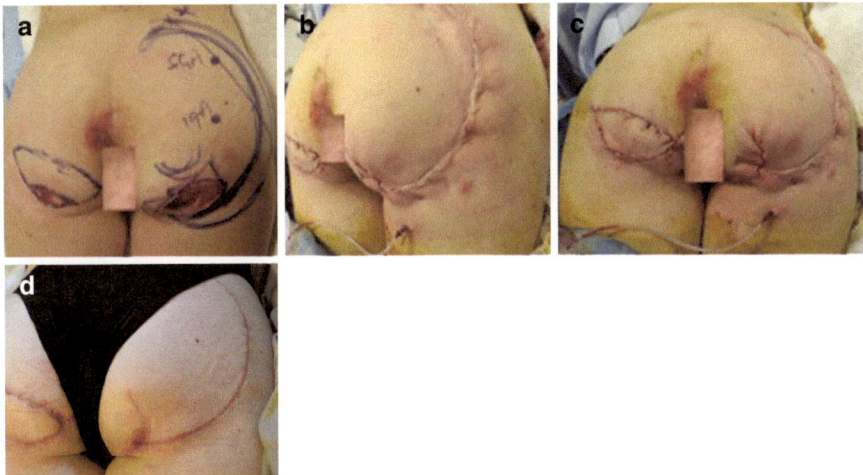

Fig. 6.7 The right-sided deep ischial pressure area (**a**) was excised and repaired with a large buttock rotation flap incorporating the gluteus maximus muscle as a musculocutaneous flap. The left ischial pressure sore was repaired with a keystone flap. Results immediately (**b, c**) and 2 months post-operatively (**d**)

Rotation Flaps on the Face [2]

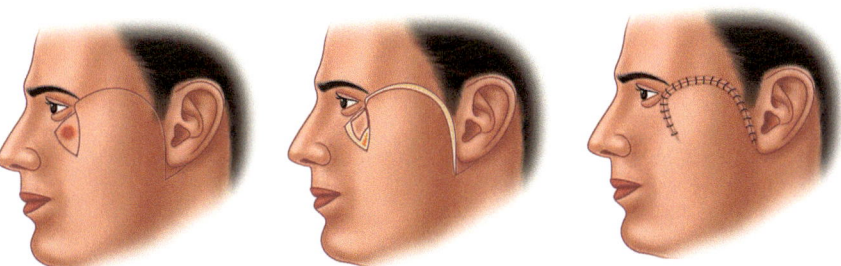

Fig. 6.8 Rotation flap on cheek

Depending on the laxity of the facial skin, the cheek flap can be reduced to less than a semicircle or can be extended into the preauricular region or into the neck to add any redundant skin as a cervicofacial rotation flap.

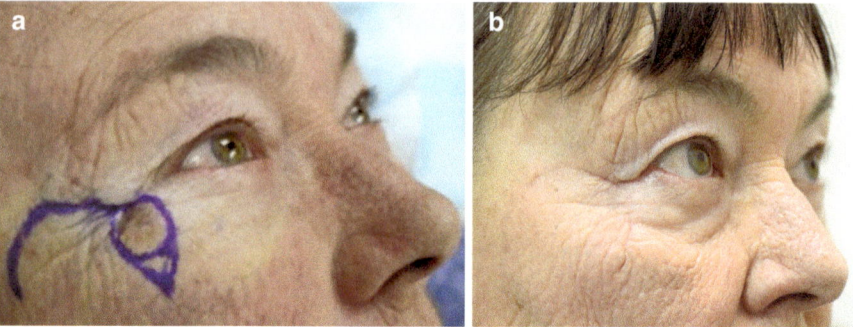

Fig. 6.9 A solar lentigo in the right malar region (**a**) excised and repaired with a rotation flap (**b**)

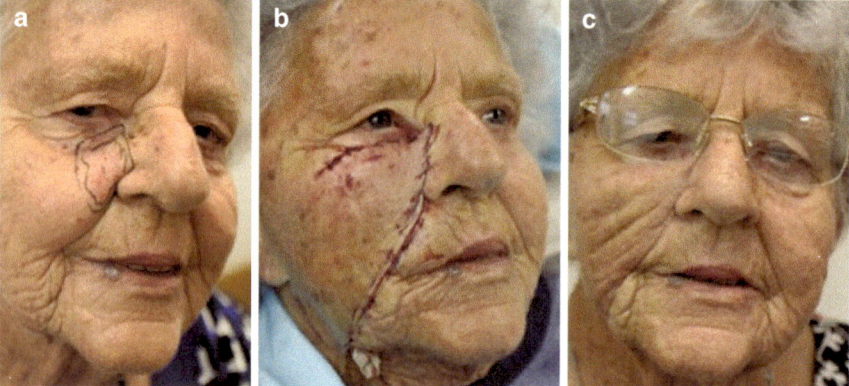

Fig. 6.10 An SCC in-situ of the right medial cheek and paranasal region of an 85-year-old woman (**a**) excised and repaired with a large cervicofacial rotation flap. Results immediately (**b**) and 3 months post-operatively (**c**)

Bilateral Rotation Flaps for Repairing Lower Lip

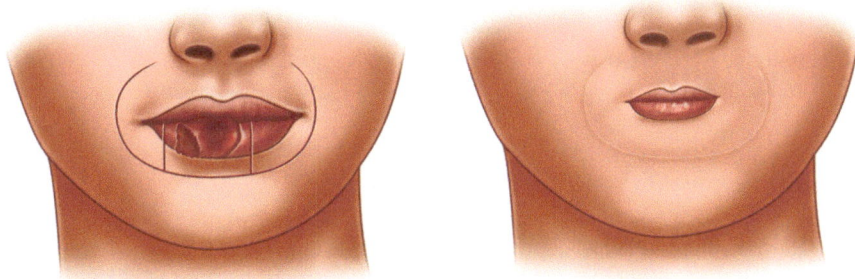

Fig. 6.11 Bruns-Chirurgischer Atlas. Reconstruction of lower lip with rotation flaps based on Bruns description 1857 [1]

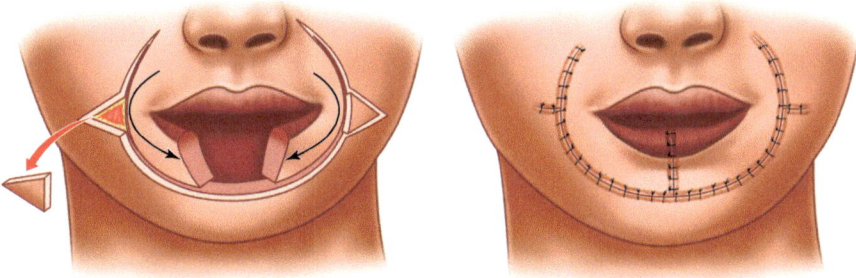

Fig. 6.12 Neurovascular cheek and lip flaps for reconstruction of lip defects by local rotation arterial flaps

Neurovascular Cheek and Lip Flaps [4]

Classification: Double rotation/single stage/neurovascular innervated flap.

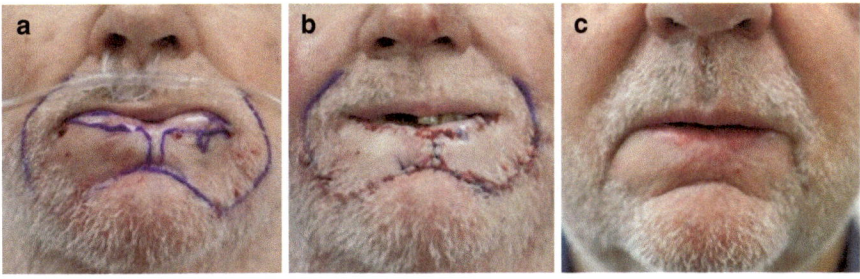

Fig. 6.13 Deformity of the lower lip with tight central lower lip following previous wedge excision for an SCC elsewhere (**a**). The deformity was corrected with bilateral neurovascular flaps, involving scar excision and release, bilateral Karapandzic flaps and a lower lip vermillionectomy. Results immediately (**b**) and 6 months post-operatively (**c**)

Surgical method: The vermillionectomy was combined with the release of the tight scar, bilateral rotation flap repairs and a mucosal advancement repair.

Notes
The Karapandzic flaps are innervated, and the final result gives good muscular function to the lower lip and no drooling. For laterally placed lower lip lesions, a single flap can be used.

Modifications of the Rotation Flap

The form of the classical rotation flap can be modified in various ways, depending on the surrounding landmarks and the elasticity and the availability of adjacent spare skin.

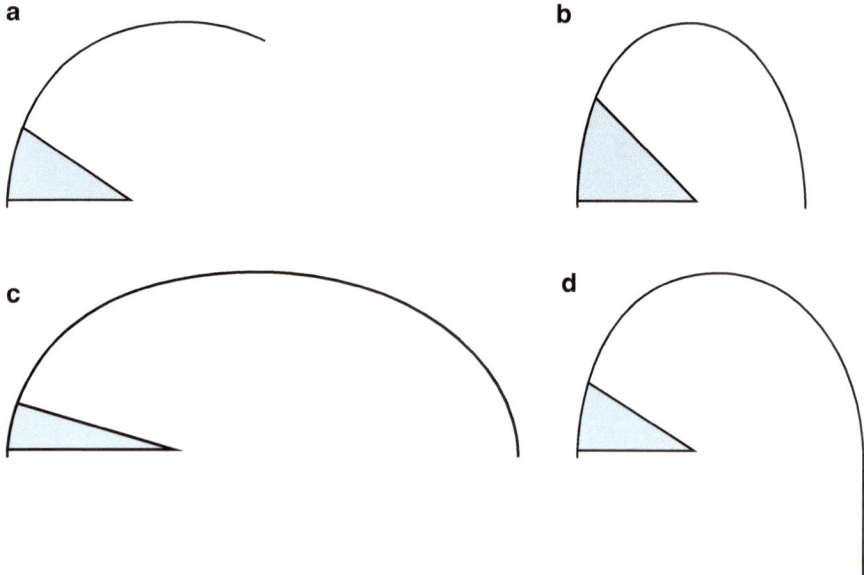

Fig. 6.14 Modifications of the Rotation Flap

The arc of the flap can be reduced to incorporate spare skin such as the preauricular region. It can be expanded as in the forehead or extended from the cheek in to the upper neck, each to incorporate an element of advancement.

The semicircular form of the flap can be compressed to approach the appearance of a curved transposition flap. The curvature can be reduced to become almost straight to avoid impinging on such structures as the eyebrows and anterior hair line in creating a forehead flap.

Subtotal Forehead Flap

Classification: Rotation-advancement/single stage/flaps that move around a pivot point

Clinical case scenario: Large nodulocystic basal cell carcinoma in the right supraorbital region

Surgical method: The basal cell carcinoma was excised with 5 mm peripheral margins, and the defect was triangulated. A left laterally-based subtotal forehead rotation-advancement flap was planned just forward of the hairline superiorly and above the contralateral eyebrow and glabellar-nasal junction inferiorly. The raised flap was moved by rotation and advancement to fill the surgical defect.

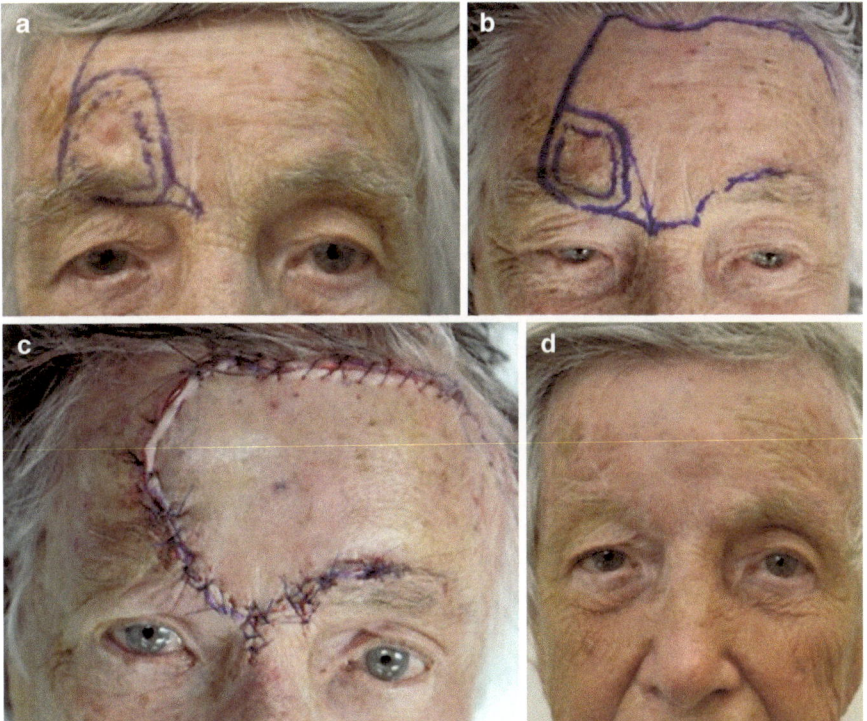

Fig. 6.15 (**a–d**) An infiltrating BCC in the right supraorbital region of an 82-year-old woman (**a**) widely excised and repaired with a subtotal forehead rotation-advancement flap (**b**, **c**). Results at 1 year (**d**)

Note

The relatively inextensible forehead flap was redistributed creating an inconspicuous scar and retaining the right eyebrow in its normal position.

The second method of rotation-advancement involves tissues on both sides of a cleft or wound [1, 5, 6].

The traditional use of this flap is for cleft lip repair. The technique can also be used in repairing wounds to reduce normal tissue waste and in correcting scar contractures [7].

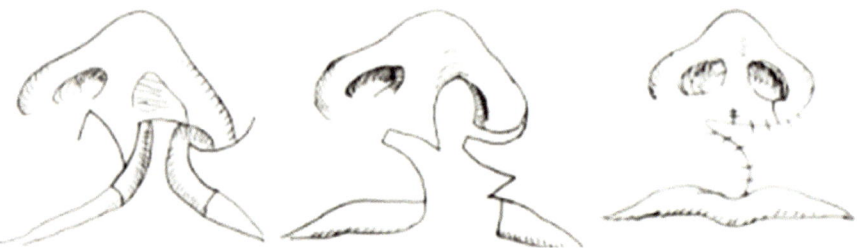

Fig. 6.16 A left-sided cleft lip. On the short right side of the cleft, a curved incision is made to rotate this part of the lip downwards. On the left side, a triangular flap is raised, and this is advanced in to the space created by the rotation flap

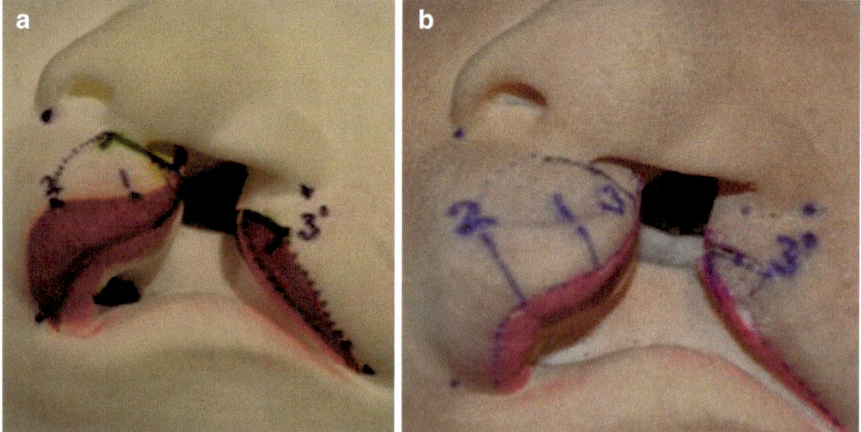

Fig. 6.17 Klaassen's polyurethane surgical simulation models (**a, b**) for learning cleft lip/palate local flap repairs

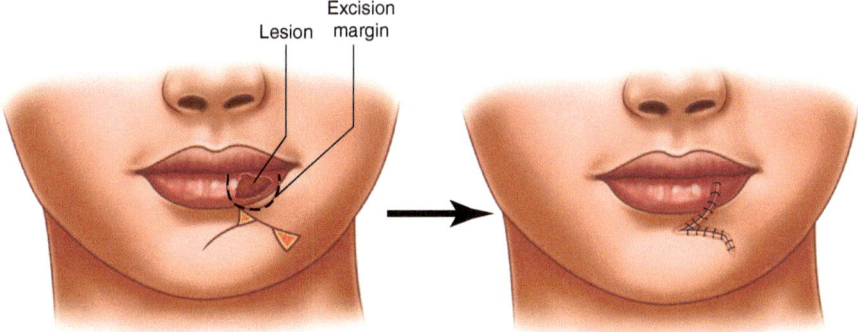

Fig. 6.18 Rotation-advancement to repair lower lip [7]

References

1. Olivari N (2008) Practical plastic and reconstructive surgery. An atlas of operations and techniques. Kaden, Heidelberg
2. McGregor IA (1989) Fundamental techniques of plastic surgery and their surgical applications, 8th edn. Edinburgh, Churchill Livingstone
3. Ahuja RB (1988) Geometric considerations in the design of rotation flaps in scalp and forehead. Plast Reconstr Surg 81(6):900–906
4. Karapandzic M (1974) Reconstruction of lip defects by local rotation arterial flaps. Br J Plast Surg 27:93–97
5. Smith JW, Aston SJ (1991) Grabb and Smith's plastic surgery. In: Little, Brown and Company, 4th edn
6. McCarthy JG (1990) Plastic surgery, vol 3. W B Saunders Company, Philadelphia
7. Johnson HA (1964) "V" Excision with less waste of normal skin. Plast Reconstr Surg 33(5):481–484

Interpolated Flaps

7

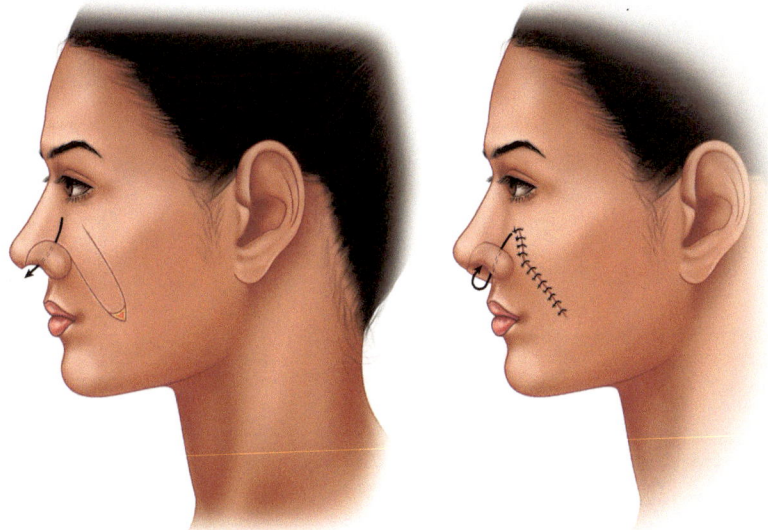

Fig. 7.1 The Charles Nelaton procedure (1881) for reconstructing the columella [1]

A nasolabial flap is pulled through an incision in the alar groove into a nostril. The flap is folded on itself to form a new columella. A second-stage procedure is required to divide the bridging part of the flap and return it to the cheek.

An alternative method is to detach the alar base, transfer the flap to the nasal septum and reconstruct the columella. [1]

© Springer International Publishing AG 2018
M.F. Klaassen et al., *Simply Local Flaps*,
https://doi.org/10.1007/978-3-319-59400-2_7

Interpolated flaps are flaps consisting of skin and subcutaneous tissue moved in an arc about a pivot point into a nearby but not immediately adjacent defect. The pedicle of the flap, containing its blood supply, must pass over or under the intervening tissue to reach the recipient site.

For a one-stage procedure, the pedicle can be de-epithelialised or converted to a purely subcutaneous pedicle. This passes to the recipient site through a tunnel created beneath a bridge of skin. Not infrequently the pedicle passes over the intervening skin bridge, and a second-stage procedure is required 2–3 weeks later to set in the flap and return the remaining pedicle to the donor site.

An island flap is one where there are no skin elements in the pedicle.

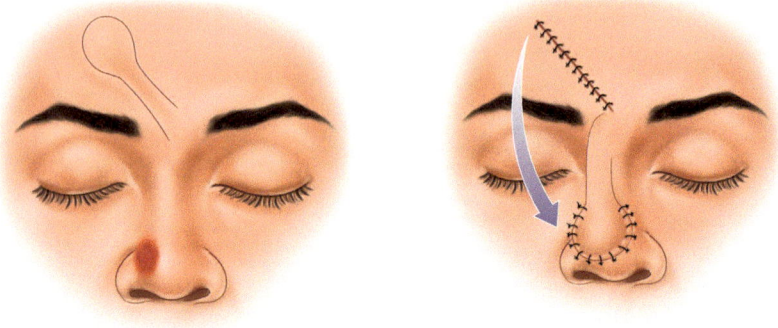

Fig. 7.2   A forehead interpolation flap to repair a nasal defect

Paramedian Forehead Flap

Classification: Interpolated flap/two stages/flaps that move about a pivot point.

Clinical case scenario: A large infiltrating nodulocystic basal cell carcinoma on the dorsum and left sidewall of the nose.

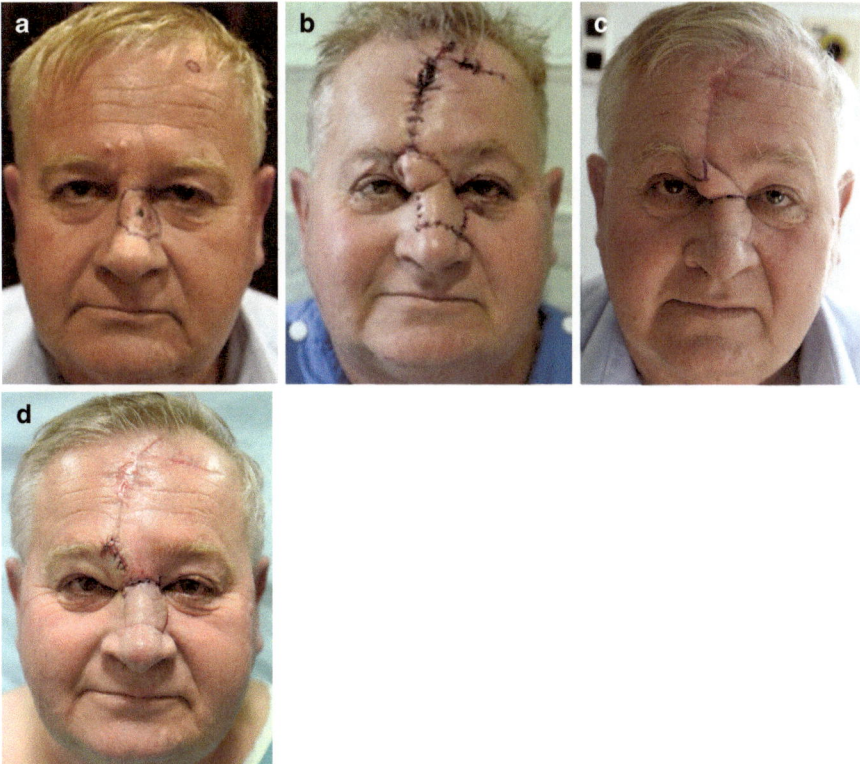

Fig. 7.3 An infiltrating nodulocystic BCC on the dorsum and sidewall of the nose in a 59-year-old man (**a**), excised and repaired with a paramedian forehead interpolated flap (**b**). The pedicle (**c**) was divided at a second-stage procedure (**d**)

Note

In this situation the flap has passed over the intervening bridge of skin from flap donor to recipient site. This necessitated a second-stage operation 2 weeks later to divide the pedicle when the flap in its recipient bed had obtained a sufficient blood supply to survive on its own.

Interpolated Flap with Buried Pedicle

Clinical case scenario: A poorly differentiated squamous cell carcinoma on dorsum of nose.

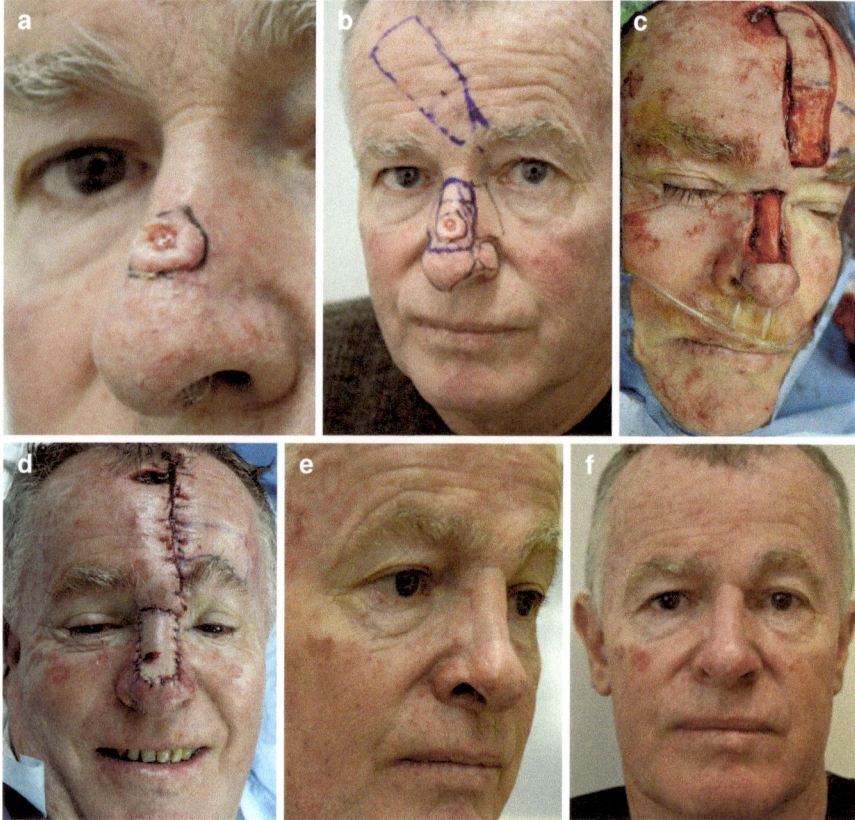

Fig. 7.4 A poorly differentiated SCC on the dorsum of nose in a 59-year-old man (**a**), was excised and repaired with a one-stage paramedian forehead flap (**b, c**), with a buried pedicle (**d**). Result 2 years after surgery and post-operative adjuvant radiotherapy (**e, f**)

Surgical method: The poorly differentiated squamous cell carcinoma on the dorsum and sidewall of the nose was widely excised. A paramedian forehead flap was planned and elevated, and the pedicle portion of the flap was de-epithelialised. The flap was then brought down through a glabellar tunnel to its recipient site on the nose. The patient underwent post-operative adjuvant radiotherapy.

Note
In this case the pedicle of the flap was de-epithelialised and brought to the recipient site through a subcutaneous tunnel. This procedure retained the subdermal vascular

plexus to maintain the blood supply to the flap. Care must be taken in creating this tunnel to avoid having it too tight and constricting the pedicle. The glabellar area is a good place for such a tunnel especially in older people with lax skin in this area.

The buried pedicle initially causes a prominence which will subside but will not completely disappear with time. Forehead skin for reconstructing the nose is a good choice as it provides an excellent colour match and a certain amount of rigidity if nasal cartilage has been removed in the excision.

Island flaps can be developed on a purely subcutaneous pedicle. No skin elements are retained in the pedicle, and there is no subdermal vascular plexus. The skin bridge between flap donor site and recipient site can be divided to eliminate constriction of the pedicle.

Subcutaneous Pedicle Flaps on Other Parts of the Face [3]

The skin colour and texture between flap donor and recipient sites are closer in composition than a skin graft. The initial bulkiness of the subcutaneous pedicle subsides with the passage of time.

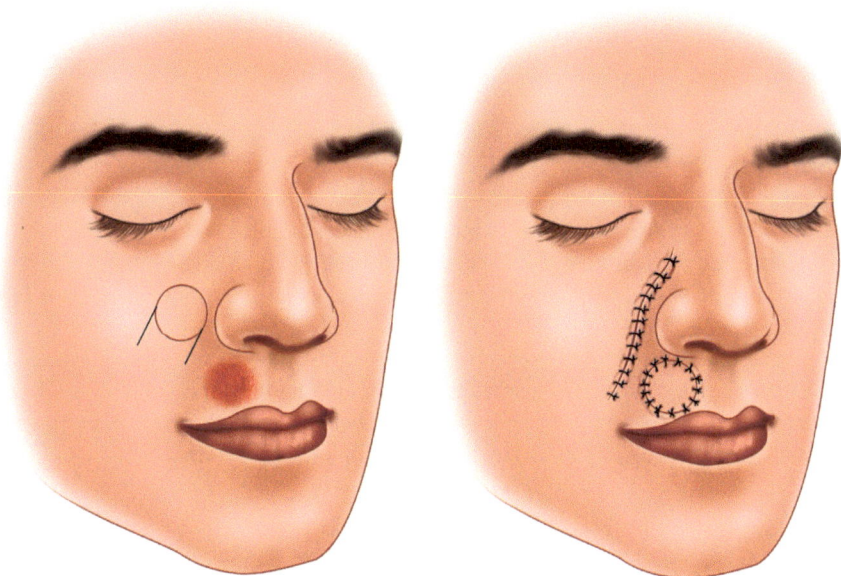

Fig. 7.5 Subcutaneous pedicle flap from nasolabial fold to upper lip

Vascular Island Flaps [2]

In known vascular territories, the specific artery and veins to the area can be skele-
tonised to provide the flap pedicle. Examples include a neurovascular island flap to
innervate a fingertip or a scalp vascular flap to transfer an island of hair-bearing skin
to reconstruct an eyebrow.

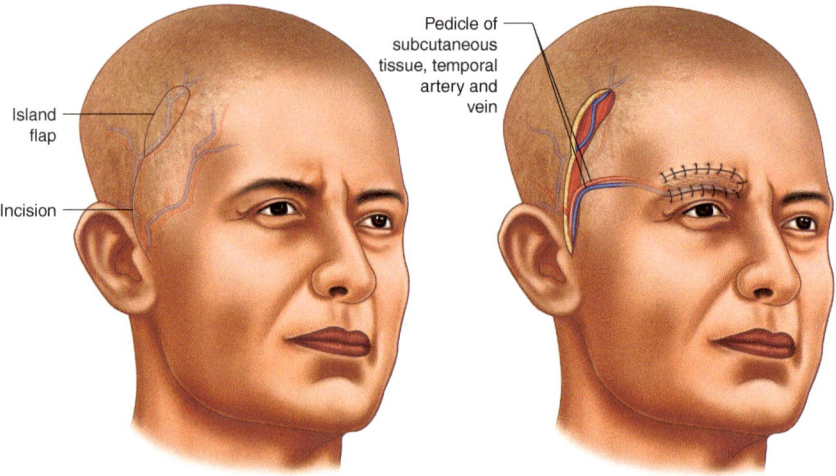

Fig. 7.6 Vascular flap based on temporal artery and vein to transfer a hair-bearing scalp flap to
reconstruct the right eyebrow

Serendipity Flap

Occasionally a flap will appear from an unrelated situation.

Clinical case scenario: A 57-year-old woman, with an ulcerated basal cell carcinoma infiltrating her right concha. She was also self-conscious about her facial
ageing changes.

Surgical method: At surgery to widely excise the basal cell carcinoma, the
preauricular skin normally discarded in a mini congruent facelift was used as an
interpolated flap with a de-epithelialised pedicle, tunnelled to resurface the excisional conchal defect. A mini-facelift was completed bilaterally.

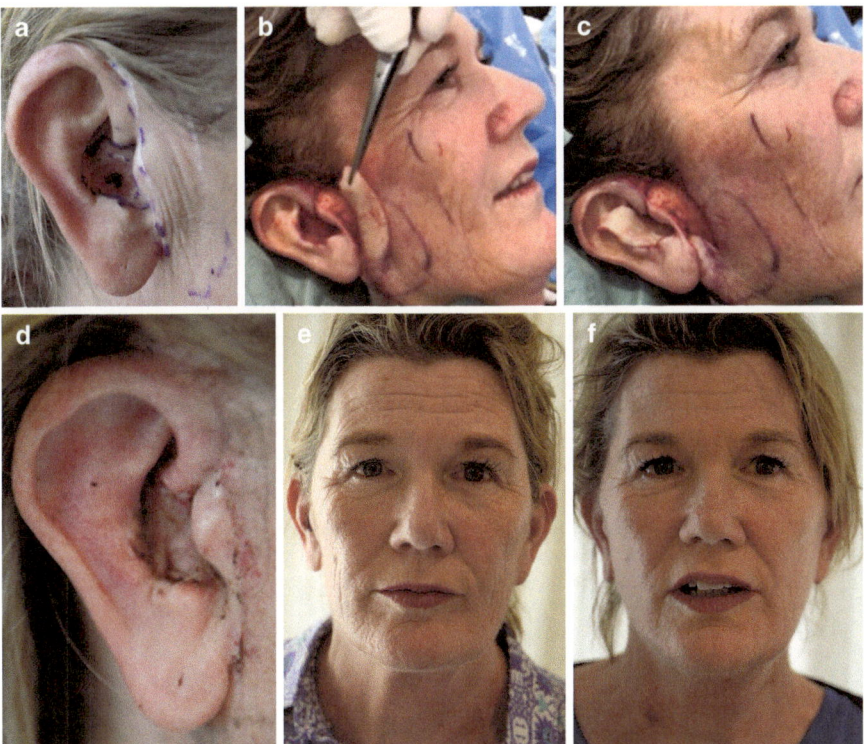

Fig. 7.7 A BCC in the right conchal fossa of a 57-year-old woman (**a**), excised and repaired with a preauricular flap raised during a mini-facelift procedure (**b**, **c**). The pedicle of the flap was de-epithelialised and tunnelled through to the conchal defect (**d**). Photograph before (**e**) and 2 weeks post-operatively (**f**)

The Bipedicle Upper Eyelid Flap

This flap, initially attributed to Tripier, was popularised by Manchester [4] for skin and muscle replacement in lower eyelid repairs. As it is transferred over the globe of the eye from upper eyelid to lower eyelid, it has been included in this chapter on interpolated flaps in addition to the chapter on advancement flaps.

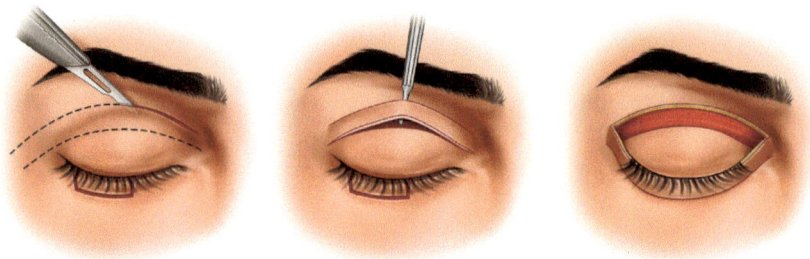

Fig. 7.8   Bipedicle upper eyelid flap planned, raised and transferred to lower eyelid

---

References

1. Santoni-Rugiu P, Sykes P (2007) A history of plastic surgery. Springer, Berlin
2. McCarthy JG (1990) Plastic surgery, vol 1. W B Saunders, Philadelphia
3. Strauch B, Vasconez LO, Herman CK, Lee BT (2015) Grabb's encyclopedia of flaps, 4th edn. Lippincott Williams & Wilkins, Philadelphia
4. Manchester WM (1951) A simple method for the repair of full thickness defects of the lower lid with special reference to the treatment of neoplasms. Br J Plast Surg 3:252–263

Transposition Flaps

8

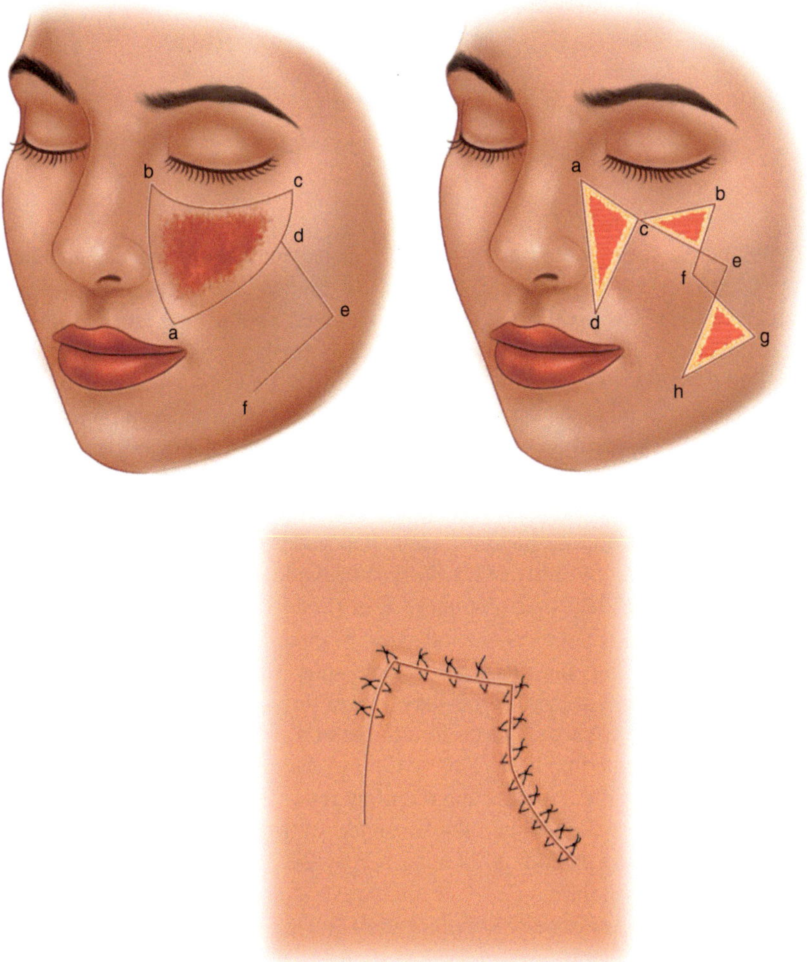

Fig. 8.1 The flap of Mideldorpf. In Bruns Chirurgischer Atlas 1857. Although described as a rotation flap, it transposes and advances. This flap could be a precursor of the rhomboid flap [1]

© Springer International Publishing AG 2018
M.F. Klaassen et al., *Simply Local Flaps*,
https://doi.org/10.1007/978-3-319-59400-2_8

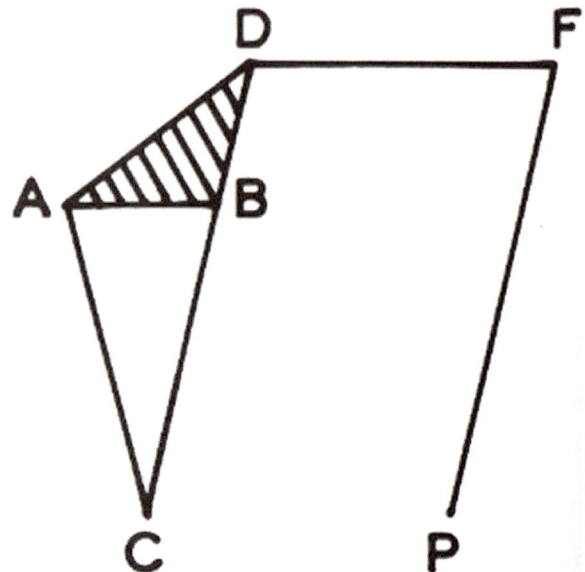

Fig. 8.2 A classical transposition flap and triangular defect

In its purest form, a transposition flap is a rectangular-shaped flap that moves laterally into a triangular defect [2]. One side of the flap is adjacent to one side of the triangular defect. The pivot point around which the flap moves is situated on the far side of the base of the flap P. The critical length of the flap is measured from the pivot point P to the distant point of the flap D, and this must equal the distance from pivot point to farthest point of the surgical defect A. If the distance between pivot point and D is not equal or larger than pivot point and A, the planned flap needs to be longer.

In practical terms it is wiser to make the flap larger than the defect so that it transposes without any tension. Whilst it is wasteful of normal skin, trimming the excess flap is preferable to having a short flap under tension with a compromised blood supply. Further mobility of the flap can be made in the planning stage by making it wider which reduces the amount of skin stretch required.

Should the flap be under too much tension when transposed, the situation may be improved by shifting its pivot point and thus reducing the critical length. Undermining the base of the flap has the effect of moving the pivot point, depending on the laxity of the tissues. A more formal method of shifting the pivot point is to make a back-cut at the flap base. This will move the pivot point towards the defect, reduces the width of the flap base and therefore reduces the blood supply to the flap.

During surgery, if the planned flap is under too much tension on transposition, elongating the flap by extending its outer border FP, beyond P, will reduce the tension in the transposed flap.

Repair of the flap donor site will depend on the laxity of the surrounding skin. It may be possible to repair the wound directly using the V-Y technique. Should this not be possible, a skin graft will be necessary.

The transposition flap has been subject to considerable modification, so much so that the differentiation between transposition, rotation and advancement becomes blurred.

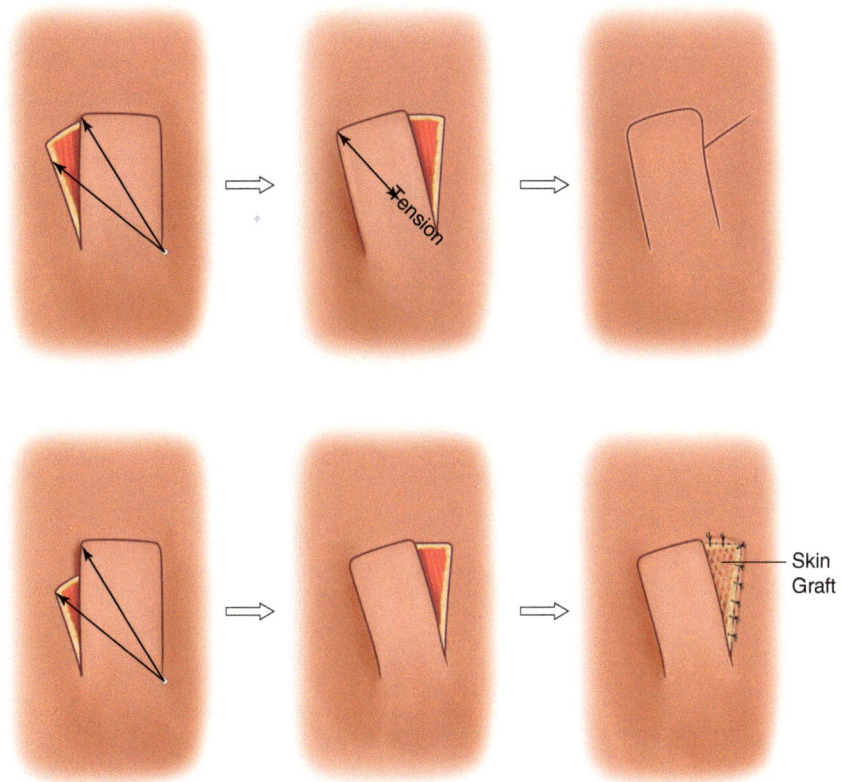

Fig. 8.3 Closure of the flap donor defect

Postauricular Flap (Inferiorly Based)

Classification: Transposition/single stage/flaps that move around a pivot point

Clinical case scenario: A long preauricular surgical defect following wide excision of a melanoma in-situ

Surgical method: The flap was planned in reverse using a surgical swab template, making sure that the flap was of adequate length. A relatively wide inferior base was used in raising the flap to maintain a good blood supply. The flap readily transposed into the preauricular defect. The postauricular donor site was repaired with a split skin graft.

Notes

The non-hair-bearing skin in the postauricular area is a great donor site for lesions involving the ear and lower preauricular region of the cheek. Whilst the donor site often requires repair with a skin graft, this is well hidden by the prominence of the ear and hairstyle.

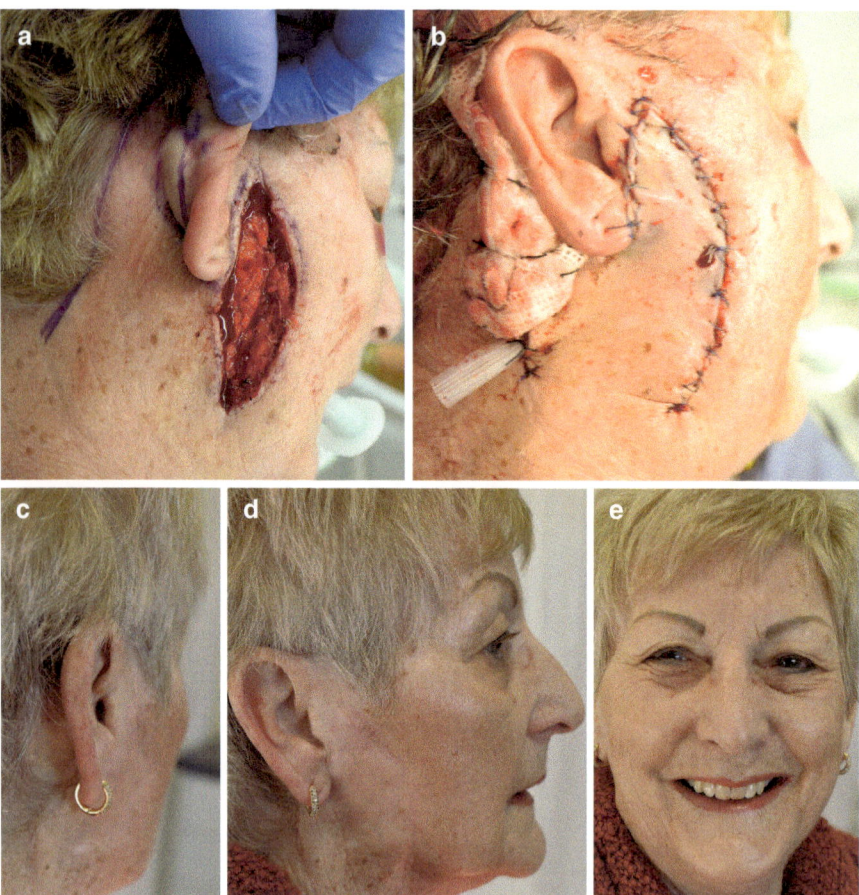

Fig. 8.4 A 6 × 4 cm right preauricular defect following wide excision of recurrent melanoma in-situ in a 69-year-old woman (**a**) was repaired with a large inferiorly based postauricular flap, and the donor defect was repaired with a split-thickness skin graft (**b**). Result at 1 year (**c–e**)

Postauricular Flap (Superiorly Based) to the Ear

Classification: Transposition/single stage/flaps that move around a pivot point

    Clinical case scenario: Defects of the anterior surface of the ear

    Surgical method: The infiltrating basal cell carcinoma on the triangular fossa of the right upper ear was widely excised including the underlying cartilage. The repair was achieved with a superiorly based postauricular flap with de-epithelialised bridging pedicle, planned in reverse and brought through a tunnel.

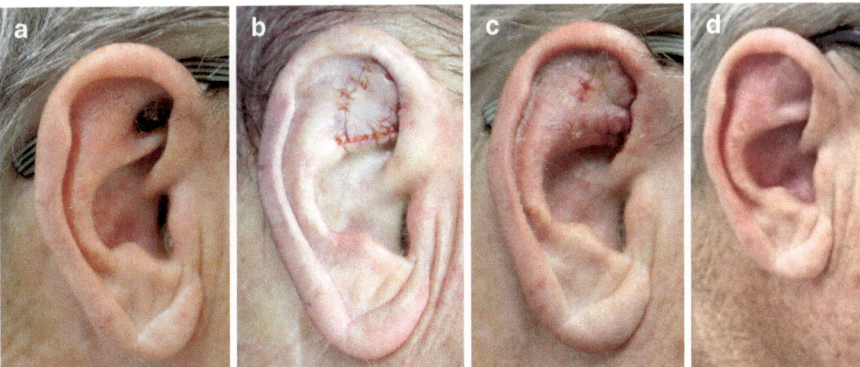

Fig. 8.5 A nodular BCC on the triangular fossa of a 62-year-old man (**a**) was excised and repaired with a superiorly based postauricular flap (**b**). Results a week (**c**) and 18 months post-operatively (**d**)

Nasolabial Flap (Inferiorly Based)

Classification: Transposition/single stage/flaps that move around a pivot point

Clinical case scenario: Left oral commissure defect following wide excision (with a 10 mm excision margin) of a sclerosing basal cell carcinoma

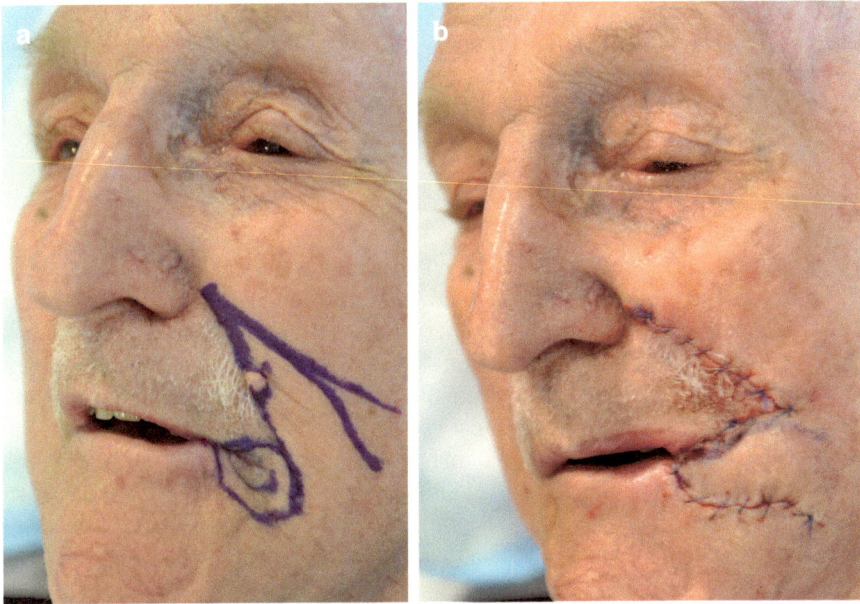

Fig. 8.6 A sclerosing BCC on the left oral commissure in a 90-year-old man (**a**) was excised and repaired with an inferiorly based nasolabial flap (**b, c**). Result at 6 weeks (**c, d**)

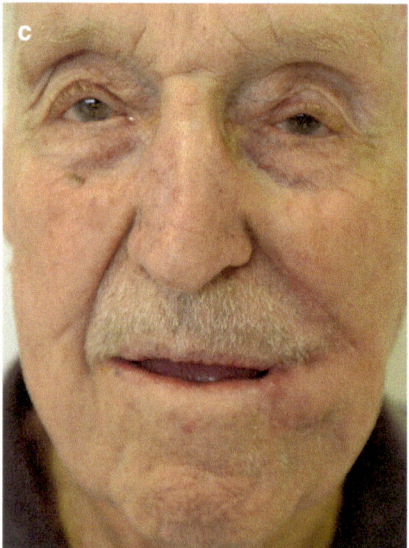
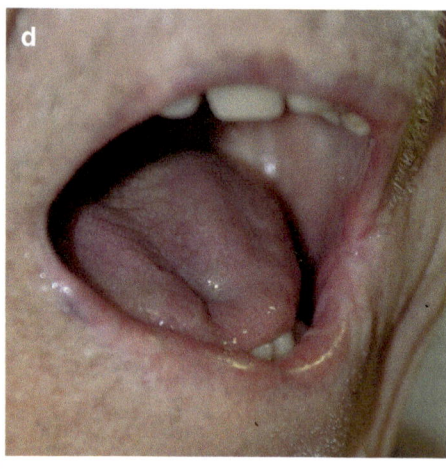

Fig. 8.6 (continued)

Surgical method: The excision created a full thickness defect of the lip into the mouth, including skin, subcutaneous tissue, a cuff of orbicularis oris muscle and oral mucosa. The mucosa was repaired with a buccal mucosal flap. The muscle was repaired to create the oral commissure. An inferiorly based nasolabial flap was transposed into the remaining defect to complete the repair. A dog-ear was excised from the lower medial border of the flap.

Nasolabial Flap (Superiorly Based)

Classification: Transposition/two stage/flaps that move around a pivot point

Clinical case scenario: Alar nasal aesthetic subunit reconstruction with conchal cartilage and staged nasolabial flap, after wide excision of a basal cell carcinoma

Surgical method: The basal cell carcinoma involving the right alar aesthetic subunit was widely excised, preserving the nasal lining. A curved 5 mm wide batten graft was harvested from the right ear concha, through an anterior approach. This was placed over the retained nasal lining at the site of the alar margin for support. A nasolabial flap was planned, converted into an island flap on a subcutaneous pedicle and transposed into the defect. A second stage of the repair was done 2 weeks later with division and in setting of the flap base.

Notes

This type of flap is prone to a trapdoor prominence after 3–4 months. Flap revision can be done safely after 1 year once the scarring from healing has matured.

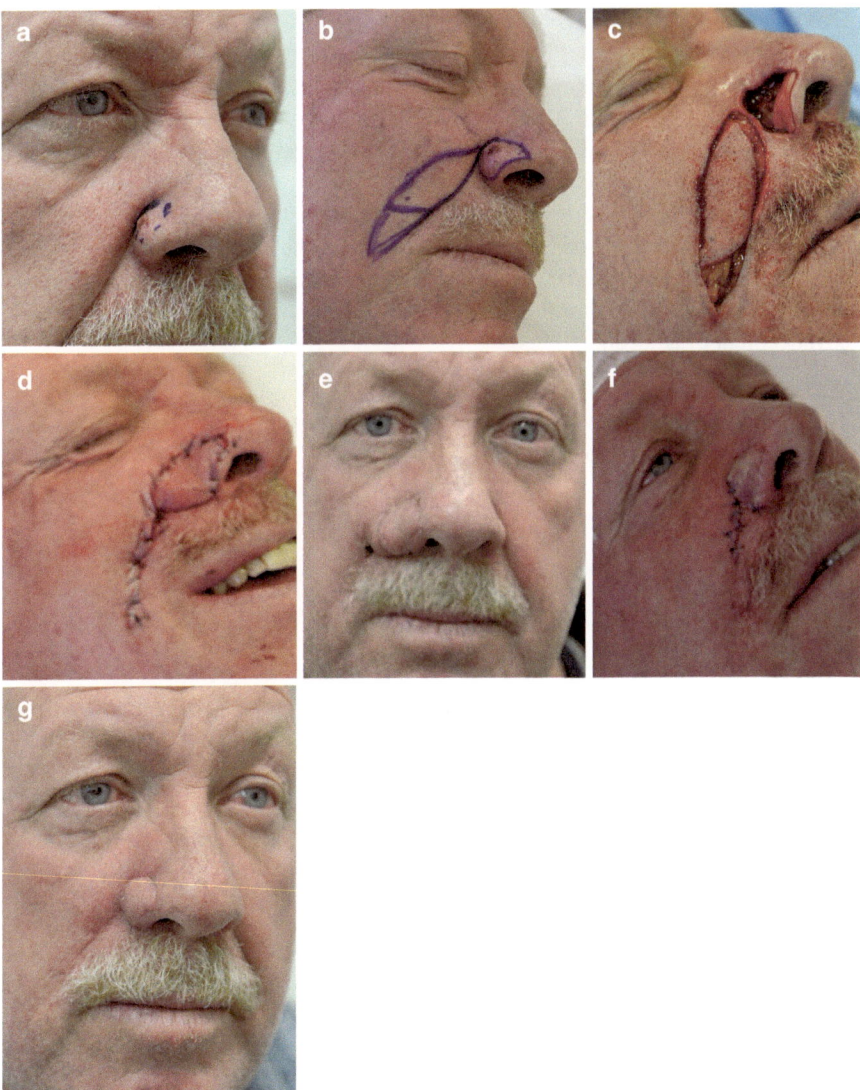

Fig. 8.7 A nodulocystic BCC of the right alar nose in a 57-year-old man (**a**) excised and repaired with a two-stage superiorly based right nasolabial flap. Auricular cartilage batten graft for support to reconstruct the right alar nasal aesthetic subunit (**b–d**). The pedicle was divided at 2 weeks (**e, f**) and the result at 3 months (**g**)

Dorsal Nasoaxial Flap

Classification: Transposition/single stage/V-Y advancement

Clinical case scenario: A Squamous cell carcinoma of the nasal tip. Because of solar damage to his facial skin, a paramedian forehead flap was kept in reserve in case it was required in the future.

Surgical method: The lesion was excised with a 10 mm margin. The surgical defect was converted to a triangle with its apex over the left alar cartilage. The large dorsal nasoaxial flap, based on the left side of the nose, was elevated and transposed into the defect. The flap donor site in the upper nose was repaired using V-Y advancement of adjacent tissues.

Notes

This procedure can be extended to include the extra tissue in the glabellar region for more extensive tumours on the nose.

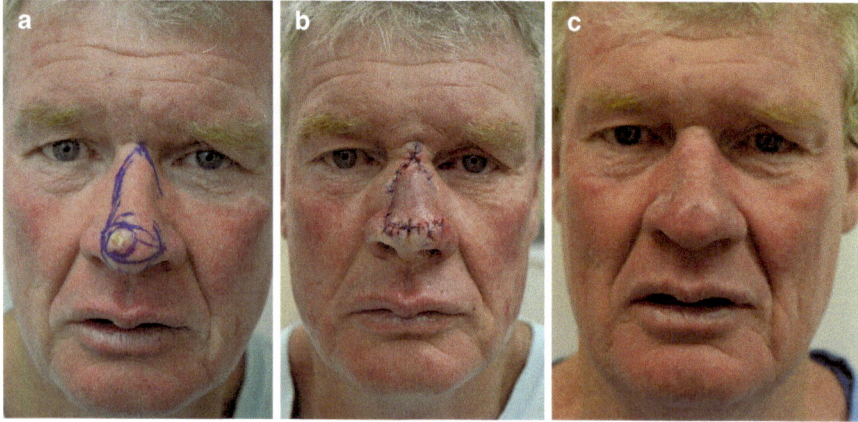

Fig. 8.8 Rapidly growing SCC on the right nasal tip in a 56-year-old man (**a**) was widely excised and repaired with a dorsal nasoaxial transposition flap with V-Y closure (**b**). Result at 2 years (**c**)

Glabellar Flap [3]

This flap utilises the spare skin in the midline of the lower forehead.

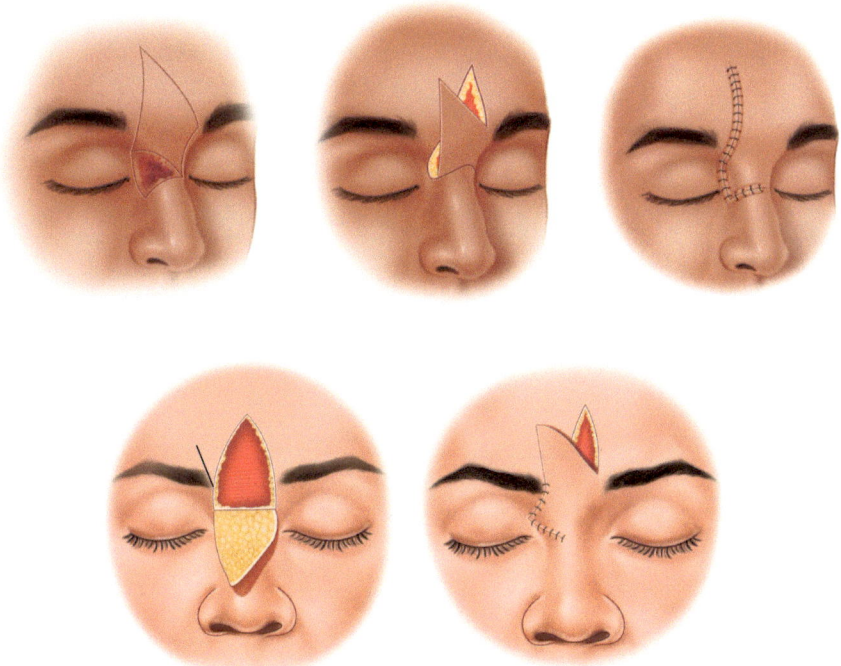

Fig. 8.9 Upper, the traditional glabellar flap. Lower, spare upper triangle of skin preserved by inserting into a back-cut (see Chap. 9)

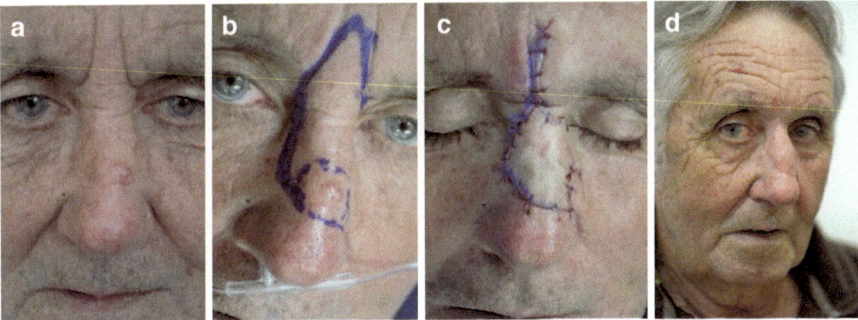

Fig. 8.10 A nodulocystic BCC dorsum of the nose (**a**), was excised and repaired with an extended nasoaxial/glabellar flap (**b**, **c**), (**d**) Nasoaxial flap result at 4 years [4]

Lower Eyelid Flap

Classification: Transposition with lateral Z-plasty/single stage/flaps that move around a pivot point

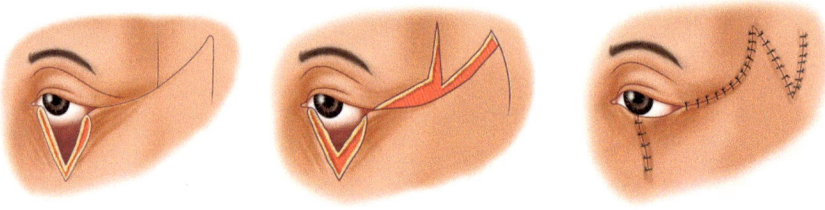

Fig. 8.11 Cheek transposition flap [3]

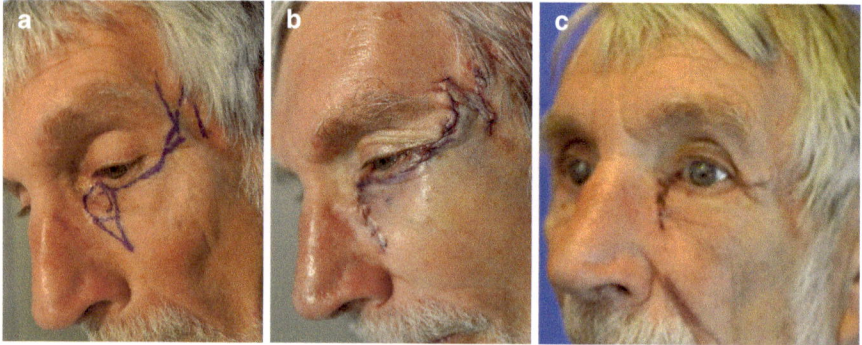

Fig. 8.12 A BCC on the medial lower eyelid (**a**) excised and repaired with a cheek transposition flap elongated with a Z-plasty (**b, c**)

Clinical case scenario: An infiltrating basal cell carcinoma left medial lower eyelid

Surgical method: Following wide excision of the basal cell carcinoma with a 4 mm margin, the surgical defect was converted into a triangle. The margin of the flap followed the free margin of the lower eyelid below the eyelashes. Further length was obtained by elongating the temple part of the flap with a Z-plasty.

Notes

The Z-plasty increased the length of the flap, retaining the integrity of the hairline.

Rhomboid Flap [5, 6]

The rhomboid flap is a precise geometric flap based on a rhombic excisional defect and an adjacent rhomboid-shaped flap. The sides of the rhombus and flap are all equal in length, and the angles of the rhombus and flap are 120° and 60°, respectively. The flap comprises the same surface area as the defect. Because of this it is easy to learn and avoids the empirical design of other flaps.

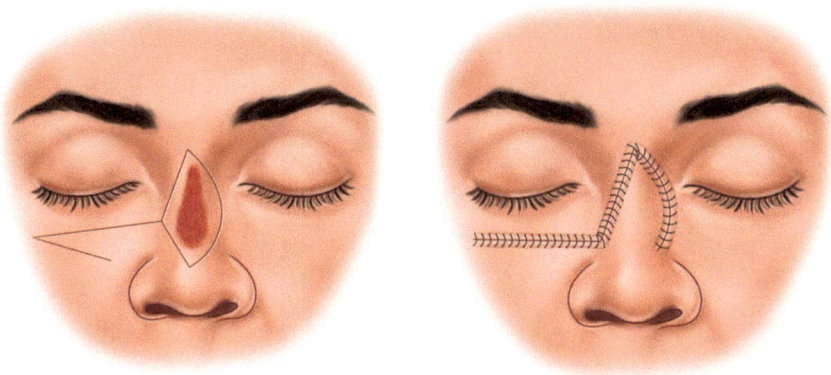

Fig. 8.13 Limberg's diagram showing coverage of a full thickness defect of the bridge of the nose by a flap from the cheek

Covering a Full-Thickness Defect of the Bridge of the Nose by a Flap from the Cheek. With only small reserves of mobile skin near a full-thickness defect of the bridge of the nose, a figure of convergent triangular flaps was used with angles of the lateral incisions of 30° and 105° and a lateral incision overlapping the wound edge. The transferred flap closed the upper part of the defect; the lower part was closed by approximation of the edges with closure of an angle. Part of the exposed inner surface of the flap attached to the exposed nasal cavity healed by secondary intention.

Fig. 8.14 Limberg's original description of the rhomboid flap

The flap is designed by extending the short diagonal BD for a similar length in either direction from the rhomboid defect to create DE. The third side of the flap EF is made of similar length and at 60° to DE.

AB = BC = CD = DA
CD = DE = EF

The flap is transposed around a pivot point F and advanced into the defect. Point F moves to D, D moves to B and E to A.

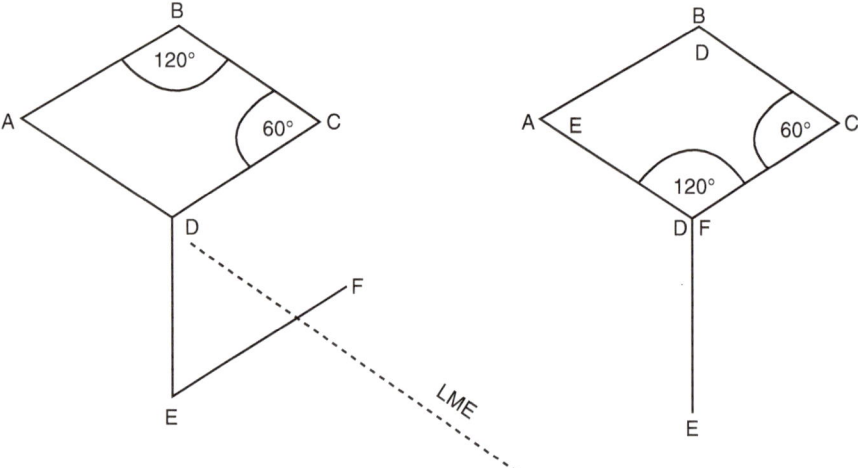

Fig. 8.15 Standard rhomboid flap

The procedure is very versatile with theoretically four flaps for each 60° rhombus. It can be used to repair larger defects with two rhomboid flaps (by converting the surgical defect into a parallelogram or two contiguous rhomboids) or with three flaps for closing a large circular defect (consisting of three contiguous rhomboids).

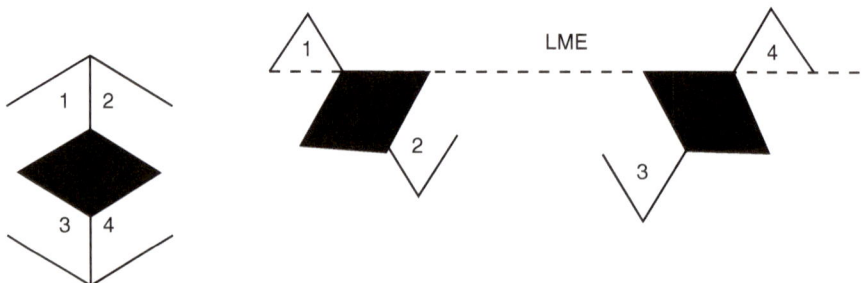

Fig. 8.16 The versatility of the rhomboid flap

In planning this flap repair, one should be aware of its limitations. These include:

1. Excessive tension—along the line of closure of flap donor site, where F meets D and at one or both tips of the advancement flap.

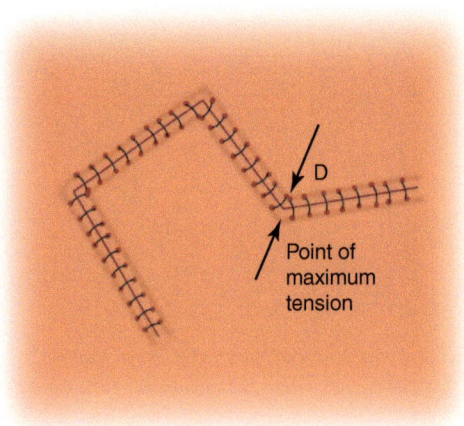

2. Anatomic landmark displacement.
3. Trapdoor deformity—tension can result in blunting or rounding of the angles of the tip of the flaps. This semi-circular form of the leading edge and sides of the flap, combined with contracting forces, can produce a trapdoor deformity.
4. Suboptimal scar orientation and difficulty in flap design—the long diagonal of the flap must be parallel to the RSTL and the short diagonal parallel to the LME.
5. Multiple surgical scars from a complex two or three flap repair.

Classification: Transposition/single stage
Clinical case scenario: Surgical defect on lateral nasal wall following excision of a basal cell carcinoma.

The rhomboid flap has been modified extensively to correct a variety of surgical situations.

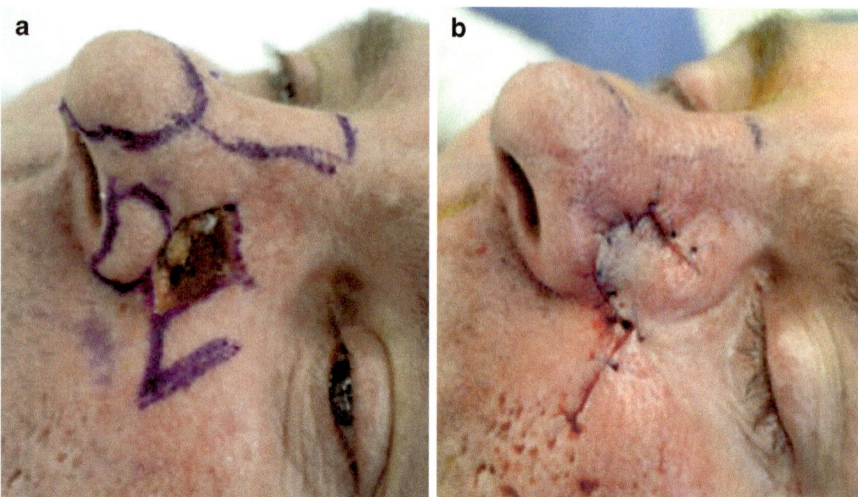

Fig. 8.17 A BCC on the left side of the nose of a 45-year-old man (**a**). The left lateral nasal excision defect was repaired with a classical rhomboid flap of Limberg (**b**). Note the dog-ear at the base of the leading edge of the flap

Square Peg in a Round Hole [7]

This procedure has two modifications to the classic design of the rhomboid flap. Firstly, no attempt is made to engineer a rhomboid defect, and, secondly, the flap is made smaller than the defect to be reconstructed.

Clinical case scenario: An infiltrating basal cell carcinoma on the upper posterior neck in a 92-year-old man

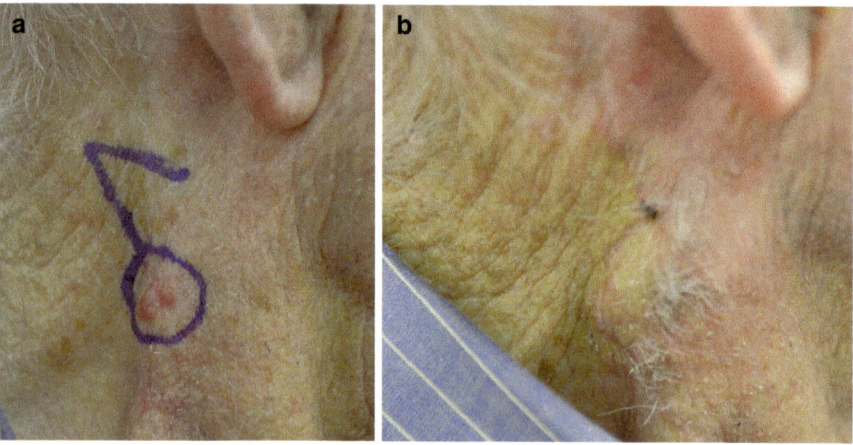

Fig. 8.18 A nodulocystic BCC on the right lateral neck of a 92-year-old man (**a**) was excised and repaired with a modified rhomboid flap (**b**) [7]

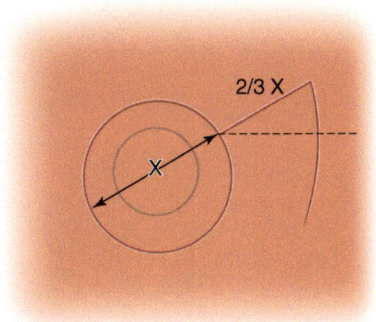

Fig. 8.19 This flap is 2/3 the length of the diameter of the defect

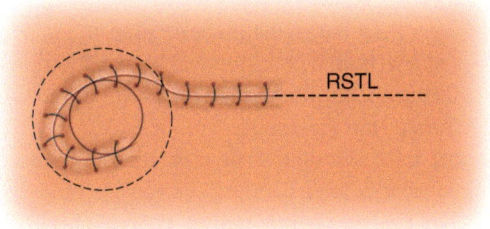

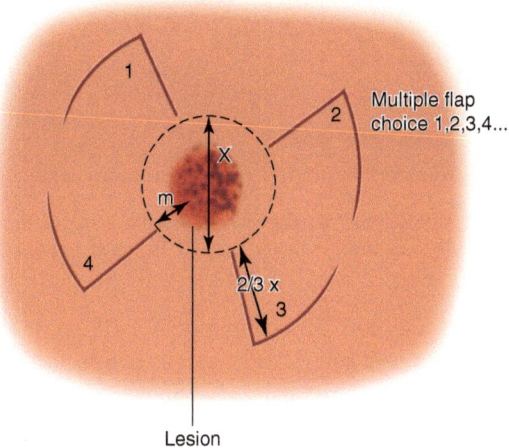

Fig. 8.20 Tumour excision margin and choice of flaps

This modified rhomboid flap has the same versatility (if not more) as the classical flap.

Classification: Transposition/single stage/flaps that move around a pivot point

Clinical scenario: A basal cell carcinoma on the left medial canthus

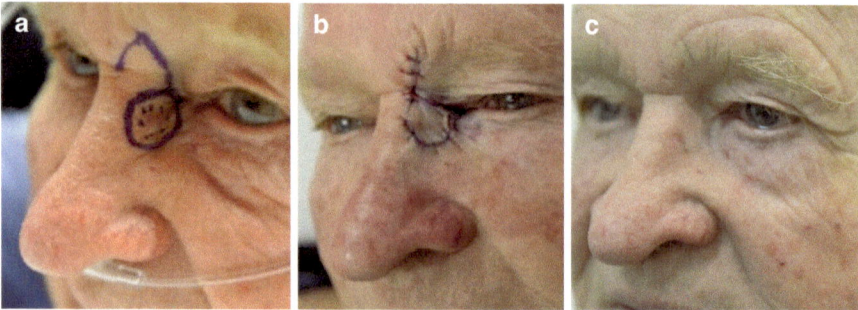

Fig. 8.21 A BCC in the left medial canthus of an 85-year-old man (**a**), excised and repaired with a modified rhomboid flap (**b**). Result at 5 months (**c**)

This is very similar to the glabellar flap.

Surgical method: The lesion was excised with a 4 mm margin to create a circular defect. A glabellar flap, based on the modified rhomboid flap design, was raised and transposed into the defect.

Clinical case scenario: An ulcerating squamous cell carcinoma on the right cheek/preauricular area.

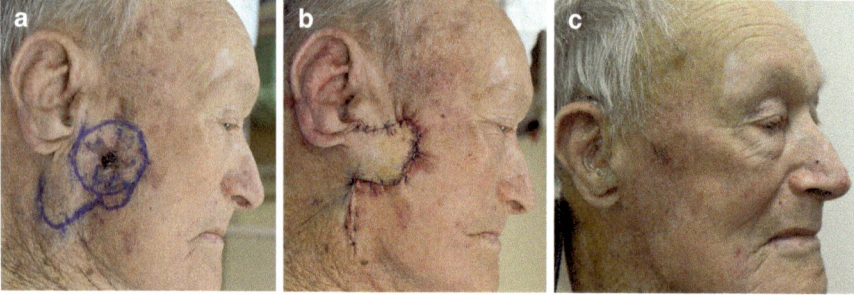

Fig. 8.22 An SCC on the right cheek/preauricular region of a 94-year-old man (**a**), excised and repaired with a modified rhomboid flap (**b**). Result at 3 months (**c**)

Surgical method: The tumour with a 10 mm margin was excised. The leading edge of the transposition flap was planned to be 2/3 the diameter of the circular defect. The flap was planned so that the secondary defect was closed in the direction of the RSTL.

Notes

Many variations of the rhomboid flap have been described with changes to the shape of the skin defect and to the shape of the flap. Multiple flaps can be used to repair a large defect such as on the back. These produce a complicated series of scars that can make problems should there be tumour recurrence or the growth of a separate new tumour in a field of solar change.

Dufourmental Flap [6]

This is also known as the LLL flap. The rhomboid flap of Limberg is classically designed for a 60° rhomboid defect, whereas the Dufourmental flap can in theory be used for any rhombus. The rhombus can be regarded as two isosceles triangles, and the short axis of the defect needs not equal the length of each of its sides. The flap dynamic can be regarded as a transposition of two triangular flaps, NQR and MNQ, or as the transposition of an irregular quadrilateral flap KNQR.

In planning the Dufourmental flap, LMNK represents a rhomboid defect. The angle between the extended short diagonal LN and one side of the rhombus KN is bisected by a line equal in length to the sides of the rhombus. The third side of the flap is then drawn parallel to the long axis of the defect MK, and its length equals the length of one side of the rhombus, NK. Theoretically there are four available flaps for each rhombus, but where the defect is square, there is a choice of eight flaps.

As the acute angle of the rhomboid is reduced below 60°, the flap becomes progressively wider than the primary defect. Little is to be gained by using the flap in these circumstances.

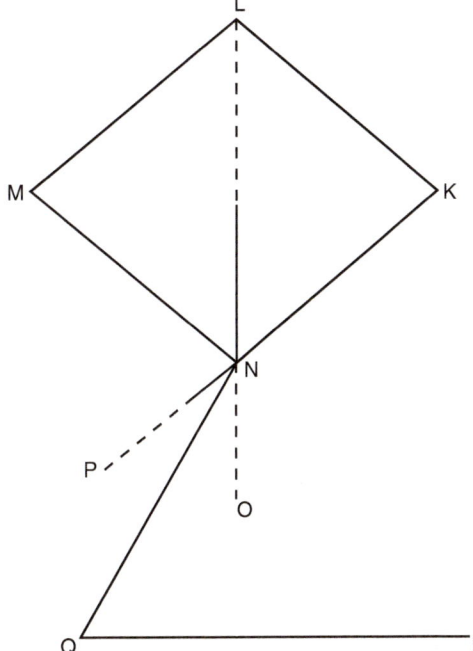

Fig. 8.23 Planning the Dufourmental flap

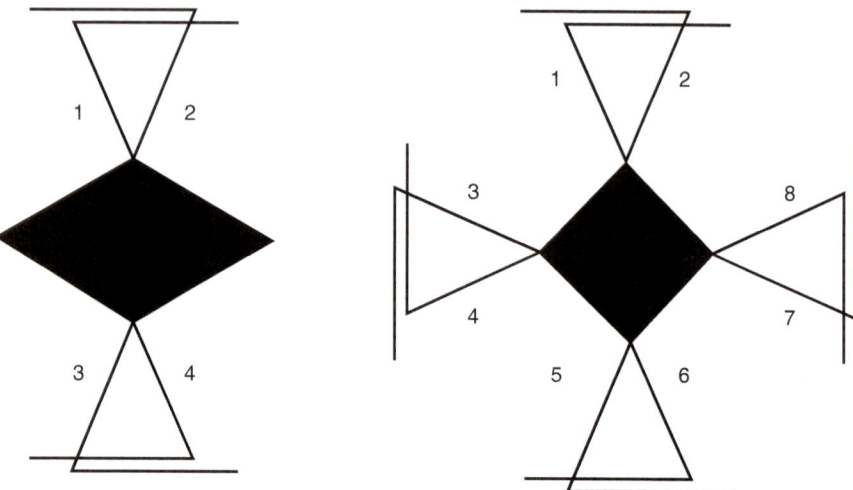

Fig. 8.24 A choice of Dufourmental flaps

As the acute angle of the rhomboid increases from 60°, the defect becomes progressively wider than the flap. When it reaches 90°, the short axis of the flap is only ¾ of the length of the short axis of the defect. It is in this range that the flap is of clinical value.

After transposition of the flaps from the pivot point R, point N reaches L, Q reaches M, and R must reach N (Fig. 8.23).

Comparison of the Rhombic and Dufourmental Flaps [8]

This flap can be designed so that its apex can be varied to intermediate positions between the Dufourmental flap and the rhomboid flap.

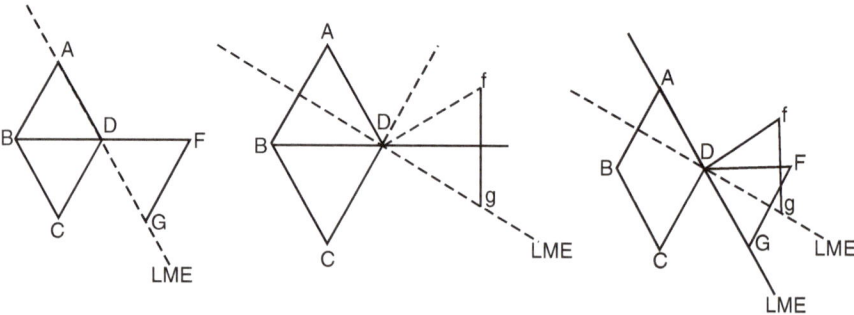

Fig. 8.25 The rhombic and Dufourmental flaps separately and on right, superimposed

Swing-Slide Plasty [9]

This local flap repair shows further variation in transposition and advancement.

The shape of the defect can vary between circular, ovoid or semi-circular. The flap can be planned slightly smaller than the surgical defect as the repair also utilises advancement of tissues surrounding the defect.

This procedure is for circular defects. In the excision, a right angle is created at the base of the planned flap. The flap is then transposed through 90° into the defect.

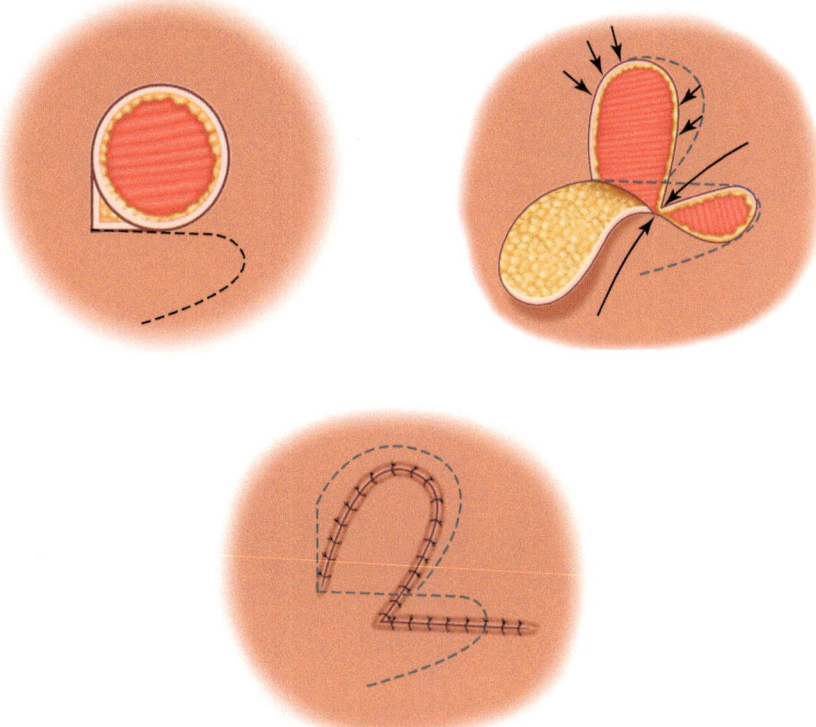

Fig. 8.26 Swing-slide plasty for circular defect

Clinical case scenario: A squamous cell carcinoma on the lateral aspect of the left elbow in a 93-year-old man

Surgical method: The tumour was excised with a 5 mm peripheral margin, leaving a circular defect. The planned flap was transposed into the wound. Final wound repair was obtained with two V-Y advancement procedures.

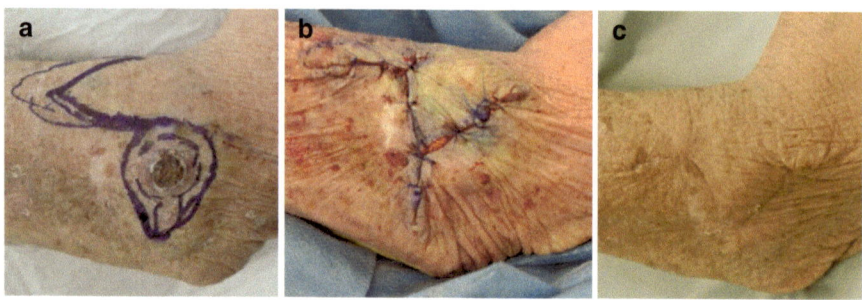

Fig. 8.27 A large ulcerating SCC left lateral elbow on a 94-year-old man (**a**) was excised, and the defect was closed by a swing-slide plasty (**b**). Result at 6 months (**c**)

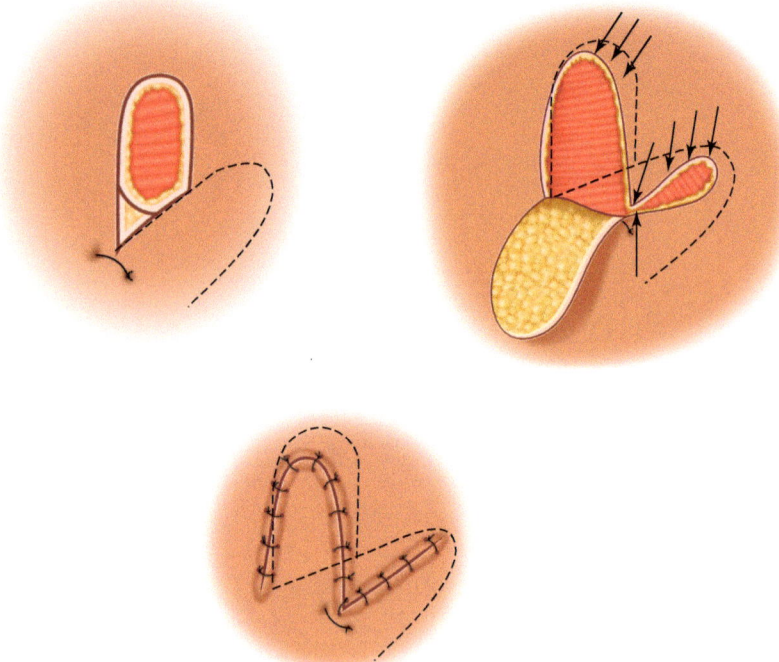

Fig. 8.28 Swing-slide plasty for an oval defect

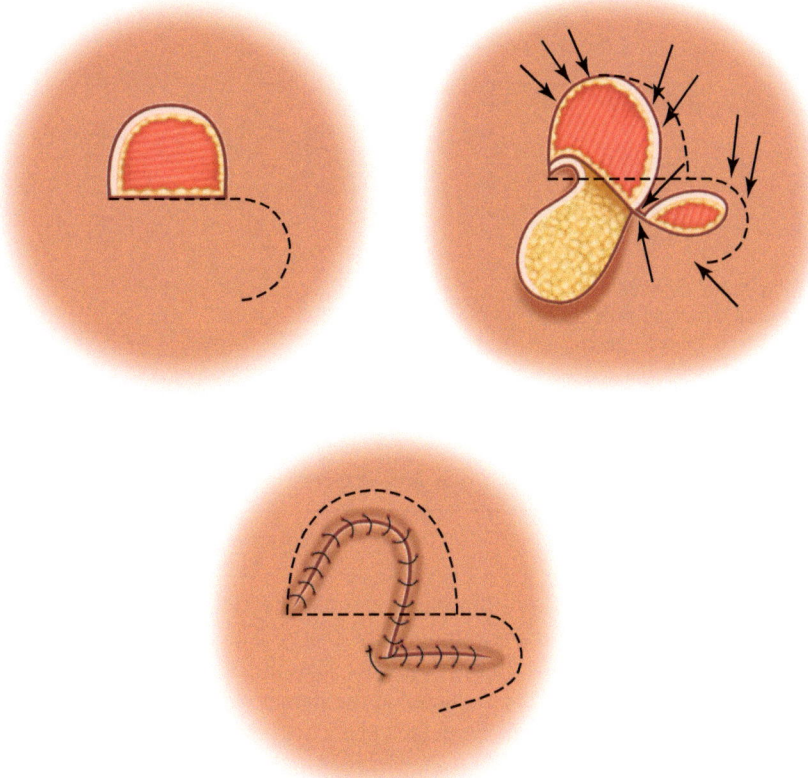

Fig. 8.29 Swing-slide plasty for semi-circular defect

Notes

In all these cases of swing-slide plasty, the procedure could be likened to an asymmetrical Z-plasty, with all the lines of the incisions taking the form of arcs.

The three models of Shrudde allow one to adjust the line of incision of the flap into the shape of the defect, whereby the flap is not only transposed into place but also advanced. The additional mobilisation of the surrounding skin reduces the size of the defect. The flap can therefore be planned smaller in size than the defect.

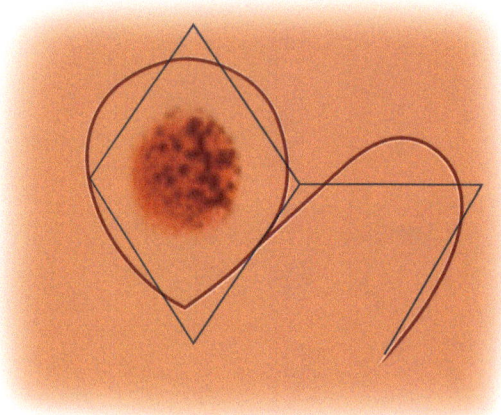

Fig. 8.30 One could regard the swing-slide plasty as a modification of the rhomboid or Dufourmental flap procedures [1]

Banner Flap [11, 12]

This is a triangular flap used to repair a circular defect. It has similarities to a swing-slide plasty and also an asymmetric Z-plasty. The flap is planned adjacent to the circular defect, its length being greater than the diameter of the defect and its width slightly less than the diameter of the defect. After transposition, the tip of the flap needs trimming to fit the defect, and a dog-ear at the pivot point requires excision.

It is a good technique for repair of lesion excisions on the nasal tip. The flap donor site is above and parallel to the lateral alar cartilage. If the flap is too wide, it has a tendency to elevate that side of the nasal tip, but this settles to normality in a few months.

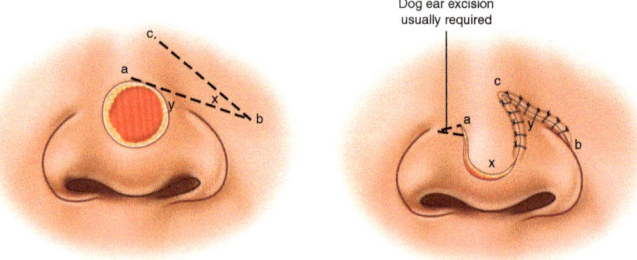

Fig. 8.31 A banner flap on the nasal tip

Hatchet Flap or V-Y-S Closure for a Circular Defect [13]

The usual closure of a small circular defect requires conversion of the defect to a tapered ellipse. The triangles at either end of the circular defect, converting it to an ellipse, are discarded in the repair. It is possible to utilise one or both of these triangles of skin and subcutaneous tissue in the repair. For a single flap, the circular defect incorporating one half of the ellipse is planned in the RSTL. A small triangular excision is planned for the opposite side.

One side of the ellipse is incised, and then a back-cut is made of up to half of the opposite side. The incision preserves a bridge of skin and subcutaneous tissue, and undermining this creates a flap that can be transposed and advanced into the defect. Repair of the flap donor site can be done with a V-Y plasty. For a double flap, a mirror image procedure is done on the opposite side of the ellipse. If the tail of the flap does not sit naturally with a V-Y plasty, a back-cut can be made to accommodate this as in a Z-plasty.

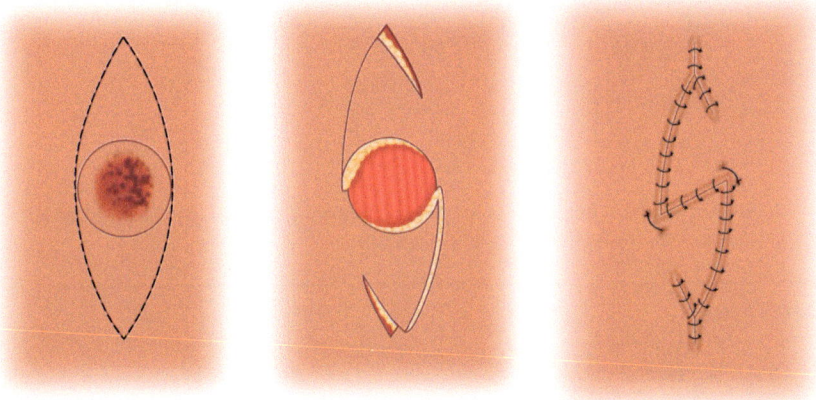

Fig. 8.32 Double hatchet flap

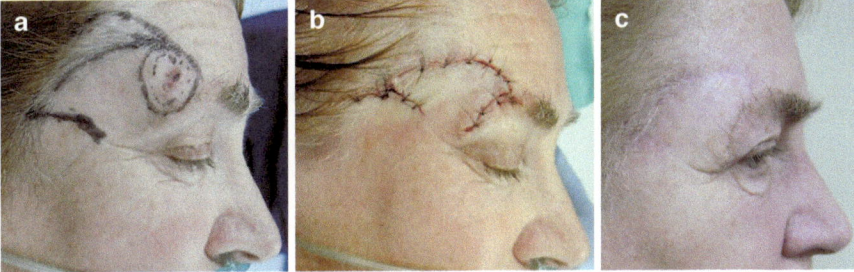

Fig. 8.33 A BCC in the right supraorbital region (**a**), excised and repaired with a single hatchet flap (**b, c**)

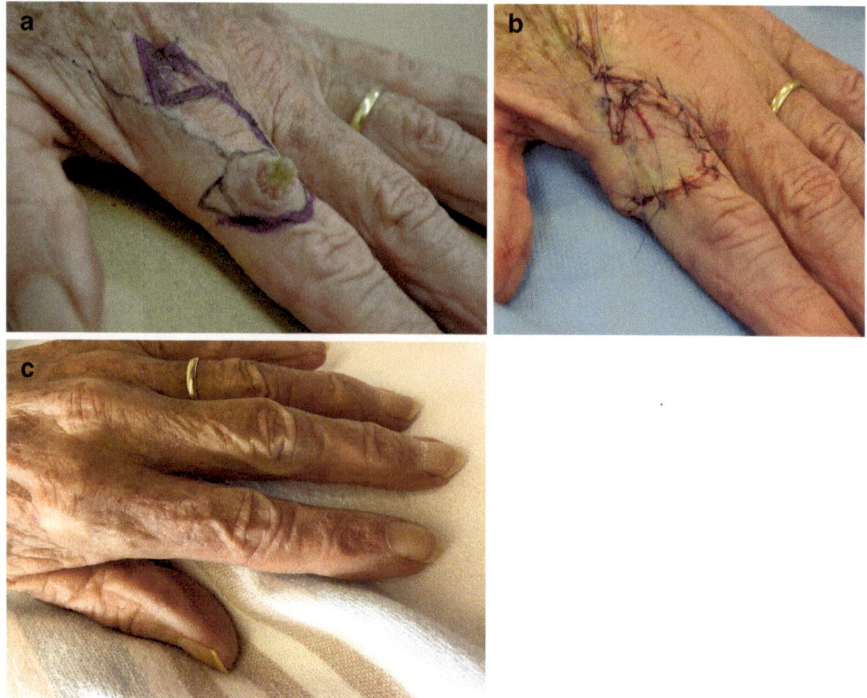

Fig. 8.34 Single hatchet flap repair before (**a**) and following excision (**b**) of an SCC on left index finger. (**c**) 3-year follow-up image of this hatchet flap

References

1. Olivari N. Practical plastic and reconstructive surgery: An atlas of operations and techniques. 2008. Heidelberg: Kaden (Olivari quotes from v. Bruns V. and his 1857 Chirurgischer Atlas, Tafel 4 Laupp & Siebeck, gifted to lead author by Professor Olivari in 2014).
2. Lister GD (1981) The theory of the transposition flap and its practical application in the hand. Clin. Plast. Surg 8:115–128
3. McGregor IA (1989) Fundamental techniques of plastic surgery and their surgical applications, 8th edn. Churchill Livingstone, Edinburgh
4. Rieger RA (1967) A local flap for repair of the nasal tip. Br J Plast Surg 40:147
5. Limberg, A.A. (1946), From: The planning of local plastic operations on the body surface: theory and practice. Translated by S. Anthony Wolfe (1984) Lexington: Collamore Press.
6. Lister GD, Gibson T (1972) Closure of rhomboid skin defects: The flaps of Limberg and Dufourmentel. Br J Plast Surg 25:300
7. Quaba AA, Sommerlad BC (1987) A square peg in a round hole: a modified rhomboid flap and its clinical applications. Br. J. Plast. Surg. 40(2):163–170
8. Yanai A, Ueda K, Takato T (1986) Flexible rhombic flap. Plast. Reconstr. Surg. 78(2):228–235
9. Schrudde J, Petrovici V (1981) The use of slide-swing plasty in closing skin defects: a clinical study based on 1,308 Cases. Plast. Reconstr. Surg. 67(4):467–481
10. Brown E, Klaassen M. Introduction to local flaps: a surgeon's handbook. 2011.
11. Klaassen M, Brown E, Behan FC. Defining local flaps: clinical applications and methods. 2016.
12. Emmett AJJ, O'Rourke MGE (1991) Malignant skin tumours, 2nd edn. Churchill Livingstone, Edinburgh
13. Strauch B, Vasconez L, Herman O, Charles K, Lee BT (2015) Grabb's encyclopedia of flaps, 4th edn. Lippincott Williams & Wilkins, Philadelphia

Triangular Flaps That Transpose, Advance and Interdigitate

9

Z-Plasty [2–7]

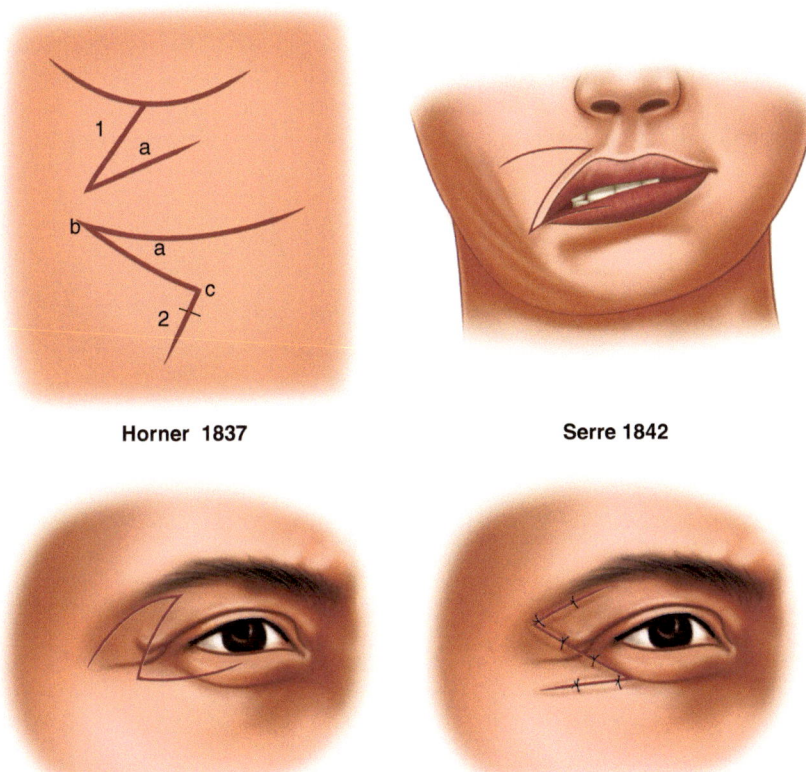

Horner 1837   Serre 1842

Denonvilliers 1856

Fig. 9.1 Historical Z-plasties [1]

© Springer International Publishing AG 2018
M.F. Klaassen et al., *Simply Local Flaps*,
https://doi.org/10.1007/978-3-319-59400-2_9

This procedure was described by Limberg [2] as the convergent transposition of two symmetrical triangular flaps. This is a surgical technique by which two triangular flaps are interchanged, one for the other. It consists of a central limb and two lateral limbs all of equal length, in the shape of a Z. In its classic form, the lateral limbs (or arms) extend outwards, at an angle of 60°.

The effect of transposing two equal triangular flaps is to increase the length along the direction of the central limb of the Z and to change the direction of the central limb [3].

In planning a Z-plasty, the basic Z (ABDC) Fig. 9.4 can be incorporated into a parallelogram, with a shorter diagonal (BD) in the line of the contracture and a longer transverse diagonal (AC) perpendicular to it. On transposing the flaps, the parallelogram changes shape so that the initial shorter diagonal lengthens to the size of the transverse diagonal and vice versa.

Whilst this is the classical Z-plasty, it is equally possible to have a mirror image, delineating a reverse Z.

There are two variables in a simple Z-plasty [3–5].

Angle size: Increasing the angle of the lateral limbs increases the percentage length gained. Smaller angles have a narrow base and smaller blood supply, whereas for angles greater than 60°, the flaps are difficult to transpose without producing cones and depressions. In practical terms the most common angles used are between 30 and 60°.

Length of central limb: The greater the length of the central limb of the Z, the greater the gain in length. The limb length controls the actual increase in length compared with the angle size that controls the percentage increase in length.

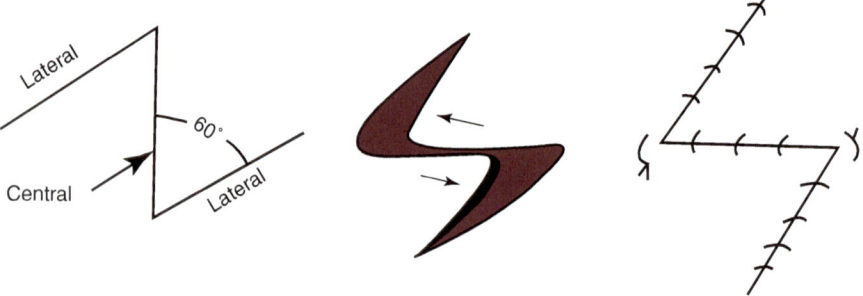

Fig. 9.2 Following transposition of the triangular flaps, the Z has rotated by 90°

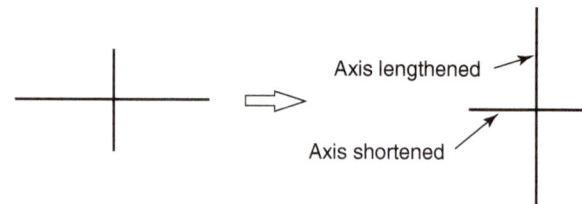

Fig. 9.3 Initial steps in planning a Z-plasty

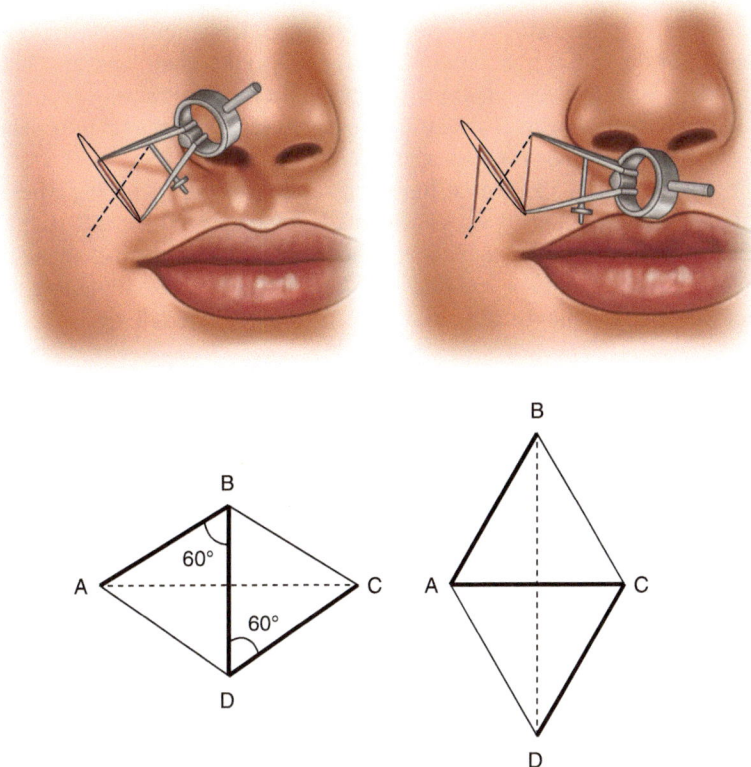

Fig. 9.4 Further planning

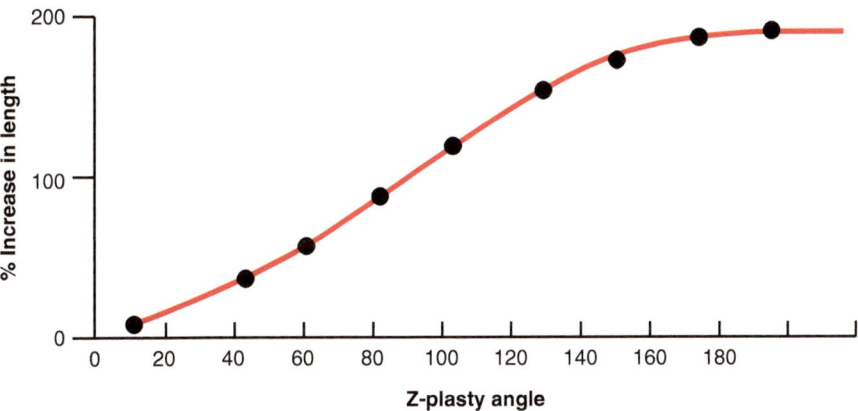

Fig. 9.5 Effect of Z-plasty angles on percentage increase in length

In order for the transposition of the triangular flaps to occur, there needs to be sufficient laxity in the skin on each side of the parallelogram to accommodate the shortening of the initial transverse diagonal (AC) to the final transverse diagonal. Where there is insufficient lateral tissue available for flap transposition, multiple Z-plasties can be designed. The central limb can be regarded as a series of segments, and a small Z is designed for each segment.

The final length of the central limb is a sum of all the segments, whereas the lateral shortening remains that of each smaller segment. Whilst this technique is appealing for regions where there is not a great deal of spare skin as in the fingers, Hudson has pointed out some limitations. The actual lengthening is less than the theoretical lengthening, because the field of tension exerted by each Z-plasty

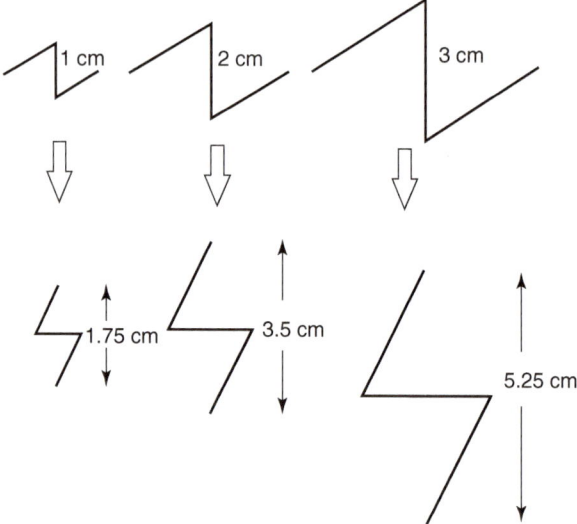

Fig. 9.6 Effect of length of central limb increasing the actual length

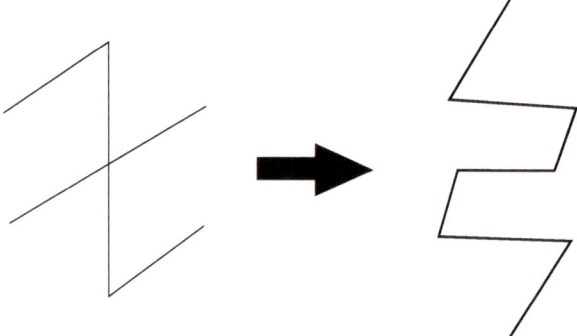

Fig. 9.7 The central flaps of multiple Z-plasties are almost square compared with the triangular flaps of a single Z-plasty

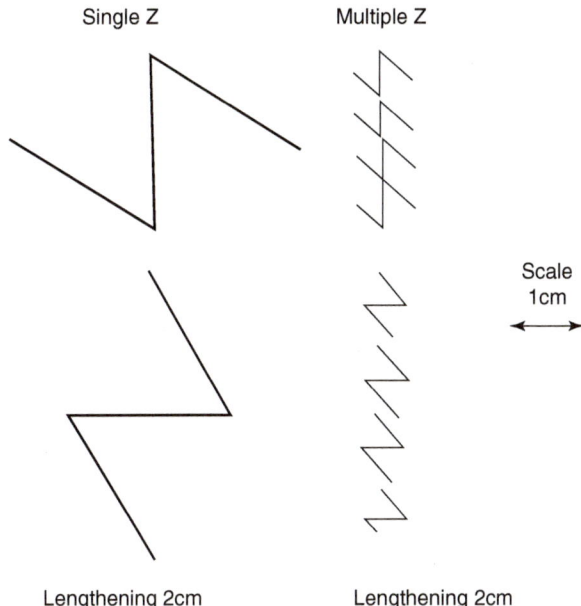

Fig. 9.8 Comparison of single and multiple Z-plasties

Single Z

Multiple Z

Scale
1cm

Lengthening 2cm
Shortening 2cm

Lengthening 2cm
Shortening 0.5cm

impinges on its neighbour and limits the overall gain in length. The central flaps of a multiple Z-plasty become square in shape and do not fit easily into the transposed position, leaving standing and depressed cones and an irregular surface. These tend to flatten out as the wound scar matures.

The functional achievements of a Z-plasty:

- Increase or decrease the length of a scar.
- Break up or change the direction of a straight-line scar.
- Shift anatomical landmarks and features.
- Create or efface a web or cleft.

Clinical applications of Z-plasty:

- Correction of linear scar contractures
- Correction of webbing, bridle scars and constriction bands especially in the neck, popliteal fossa, axilla and digits
- Release of circular contractures around body orifices, e.g. nostril, ear and mouth.
- As a planned procedure to avoid scar contractures or change the direction of scars (as in release of Dupuytren's contracture)
- As an adjunct to closing surgical wounds

Classification: Double-opposing transposition/single stage/flaps that move about a pivot point

Clinical case scenario: Unsightly tracheostomy scar with vertical orientation

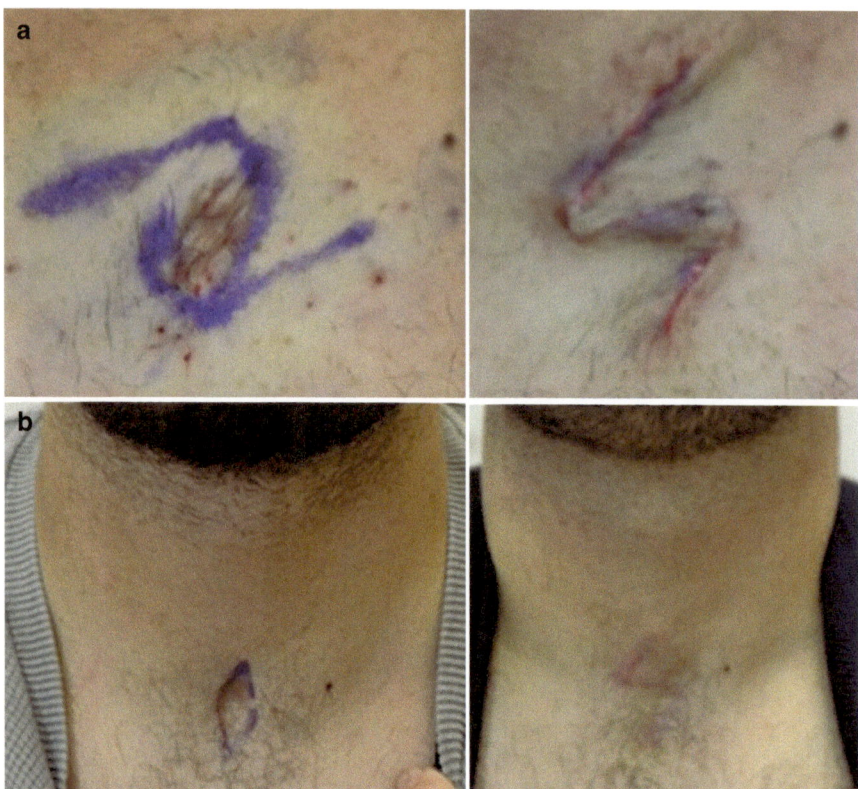

Fig. 9.9 Revision of a vertical tracheostomy scar with a Z-plasty revision in a 30-year-old man after major trauma (**a**). Result at 4 months (**b**)

Surgical method: A Z-plasty was planned to incorporate the vertical scar as the central limb. After excising the scar and transposing the triangular flaps, the central limb of the Z was oriented horizontally in the relaxed skin tension line.

Notes

Unless in an extreme emergency, vertical tracheostomy incisions should be avoided. They always leave unsightly scars that are difficult to disguise.

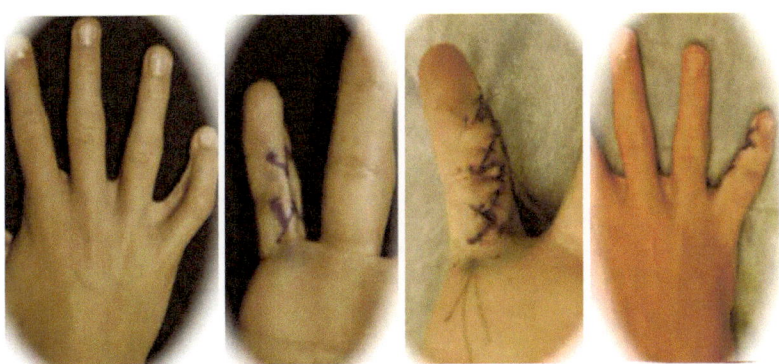

Fig. 9.10 Multiple Z-plasties to correct a contracture of the right little finger

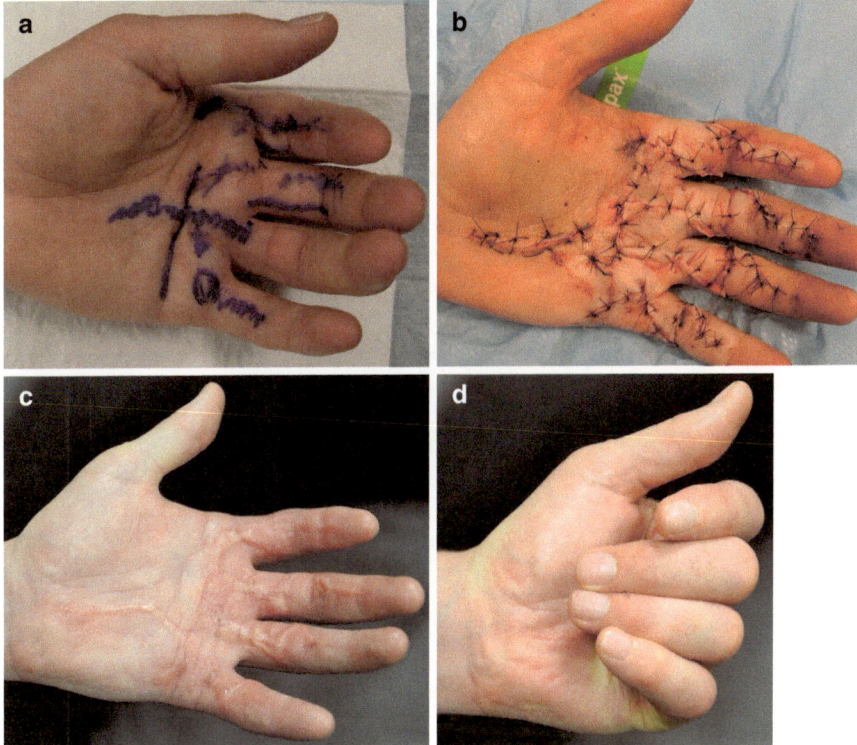

Fig. 9.11 Multiple single Z-plasties as commonly used in Dupuytren's contracture release at the bases of index, middle, ring and little fingers. Recurrent severe Dupuytren's fibromatosis in a left-hand dominant 48-year-old man (**a**). First post-operative day (**b**) and result at 10 weeks (**c, d**)

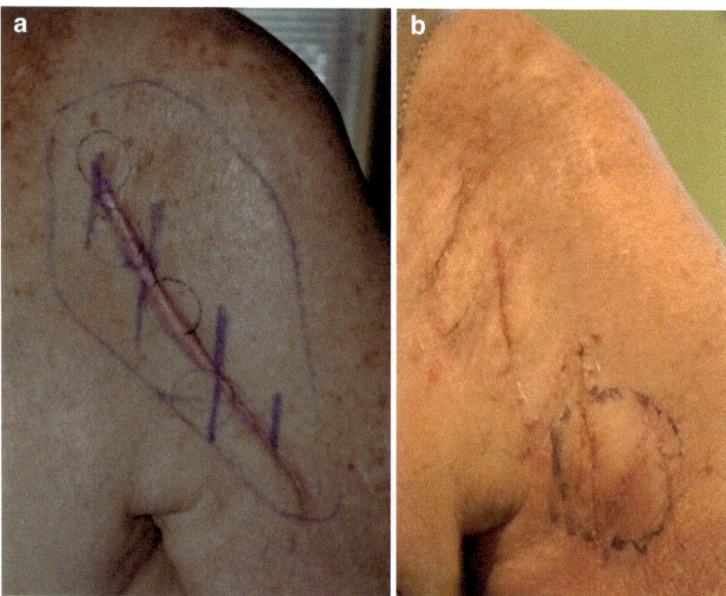

Fig. 9.12 A painful keloid scar on the left shoulder following arthroplasty in a 65-year-old woman (**a**). Released with multiple Z-plasties (**b**)

Z-plasties in this situation give an accordion like elasticity and insert additional skin along the longitudinal axis of the joint.

Planning a Scar Revision on the Face

The intended line of the transverse limb of the Z-plasty follows the resting skin tension line.

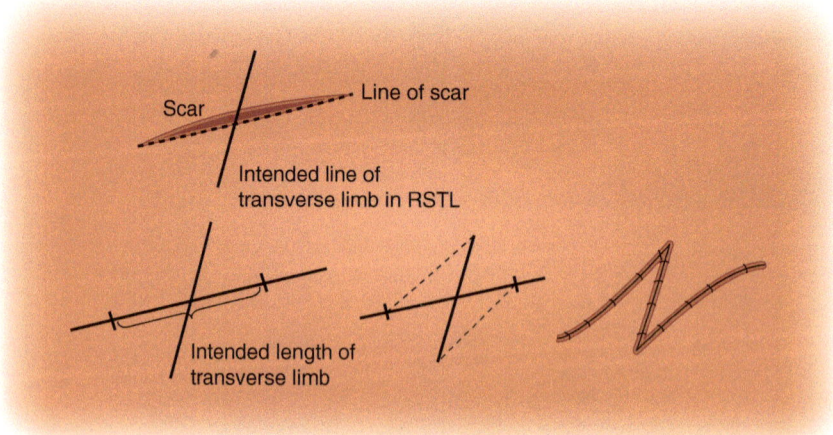

Fig. 9.13 Changing the direction of a scar. See Fig 9.4 The central limb of the transposed triangular flaps is now in the RSTL

Planning Z-Plasties in Three Dimensions

Planning is simplified by assessing the problem in two dimensions, one axis being too long and requiring reduction and the other axis too short and requiring lengthening.

Notching of the Lip

The axes to be considered are the line of the notch and the line of the lip margin. They are perpendicular to each other. The line of the notch can be considered too short and the line of the lip margin, too long. A Z-plasty will therefore shorten one axis and lengthen the other.

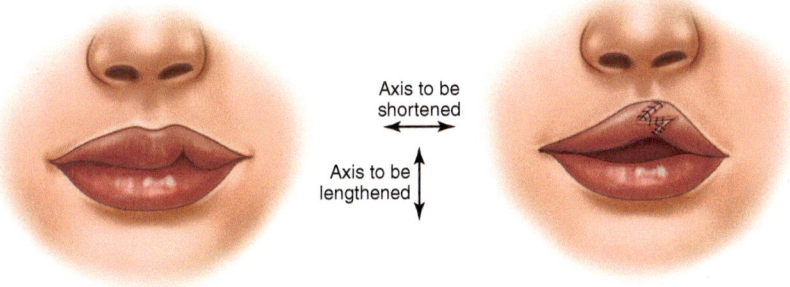

Fig. 9.14 Analysis of a notch in the upper lip

Bridle Scar

The axes to be considered are the line of the scar itself and a line drawn at right angles to it.

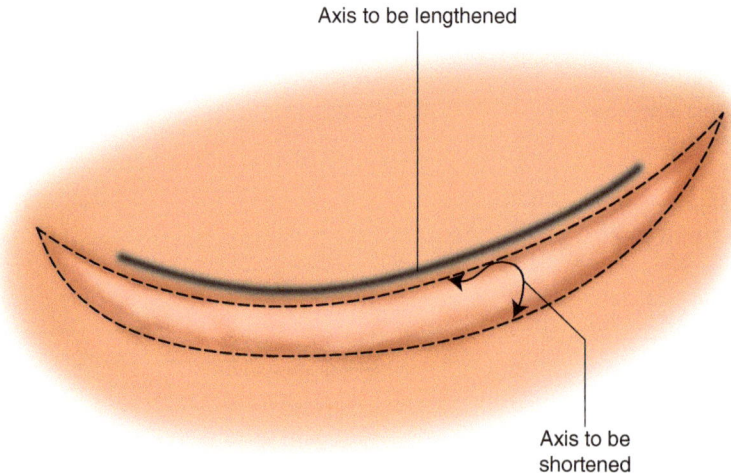

Axis to be lengthened

Axis to be
shortened

Fig. 9.15 Analysis of bridle scar

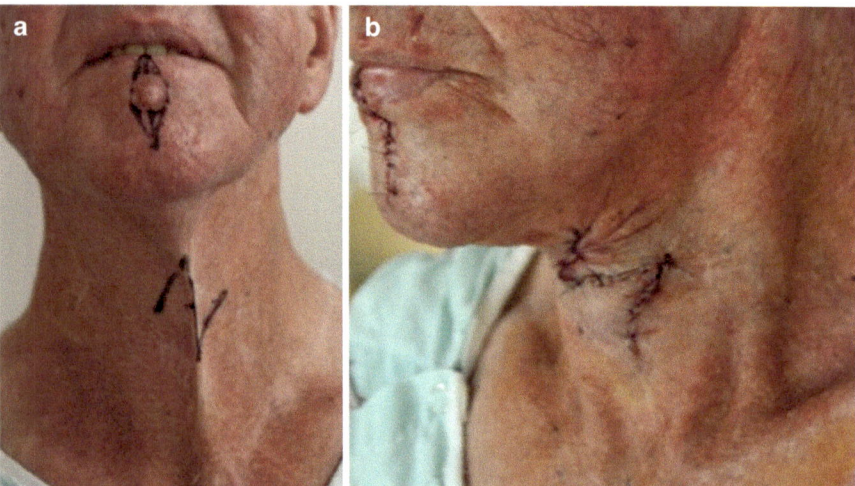

Fig. 9.16 A bridle scar contracture of the anterior neck resulting from previous cancer excision
(**a**), released by a Z-plasty (**b**)

Congenital Ring Constriction

The circumference of the limb at the base of the constriction can be regarded as the
short axis. The depression into the constriction, an axis at right angles to the former,
is too long. Whilst this type of correction is frequently published in plastic surgery
texts, in our experience the final results are disappointing.

Fig. 9.17 Correcting a
congenital ring constriction

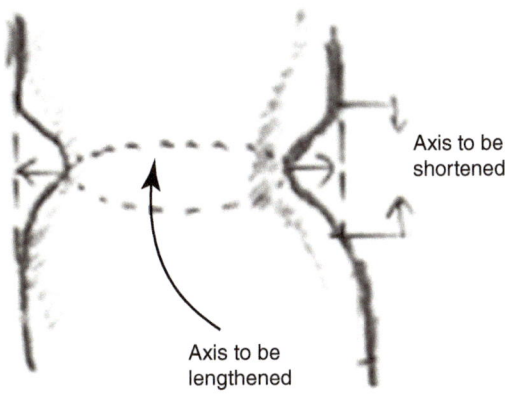

Modifying the Z-Plasty Flaps

The tips of the flaps can be broadened to improve their vascularity. The transposed flaps, however, do not fit well into the adjacent defects.

Fig. 9.18 Modifying the
flap shape [3]

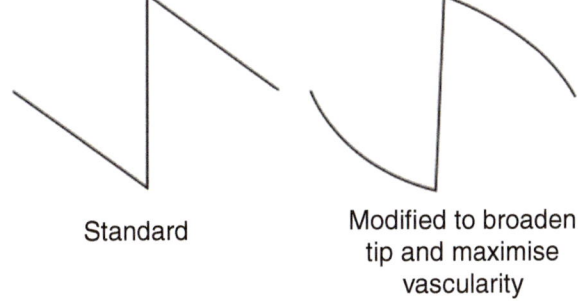

Tetrahedral Z-Plasty

In the creation or obliteration of a cleft or web by Z-plasty, four plane surfaces are involved. Two planes are occupied by two triangular flaps in their initial position, and two other planes are occupied by flaps in their transposed position. These four planes intersect to form a four-sided figure or tetrahedron.

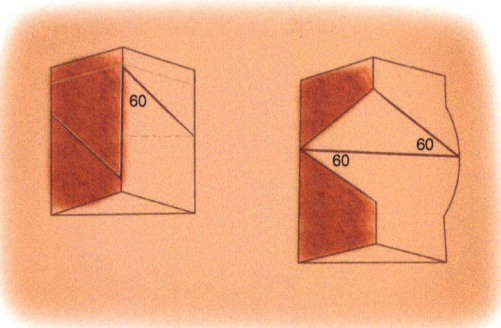

Fig. 9.19 Planning a tetrahedral Z-plasty

Finger Web

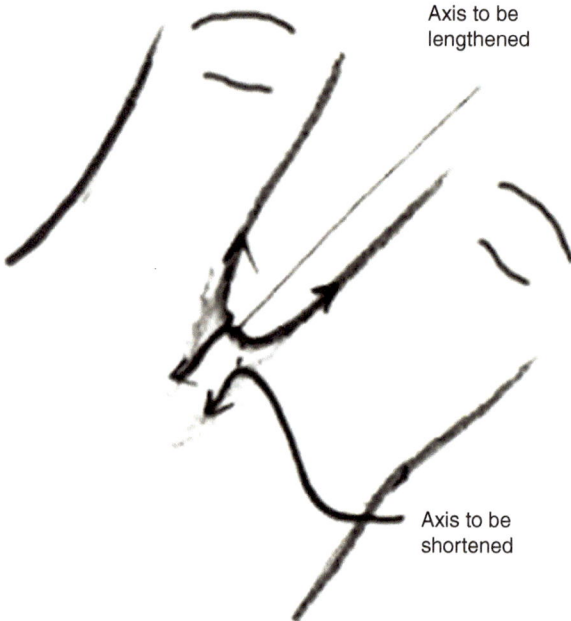

Fig. 9.20 The line of the web needs to be lengthened, and the line in the opposite axis needs to be shortened in order to deepen the web

Asymmetrical Z-Plasty

This procedure is useful when local features such as the scalp hairline, dense scar tissue or other anatomical features hinder the use of a symmetrical Z-plasty. It is planned with different angles, one of which can be 90° and the other considerably smaller. The flap with the narrowest angle is the most mobile, and with a narrower base, more transposition can be achieved. This narrower flap has a greater tendency towards a dog-ear since it moves through a greater arc and closes a larger angle. The increase in length and decrease in breadth of the procedure following transposition occur mainly around the base of the narrower flap. As the angle of the broader flap increases, its mobility decreases, and finally an end point is reached where it does not move.

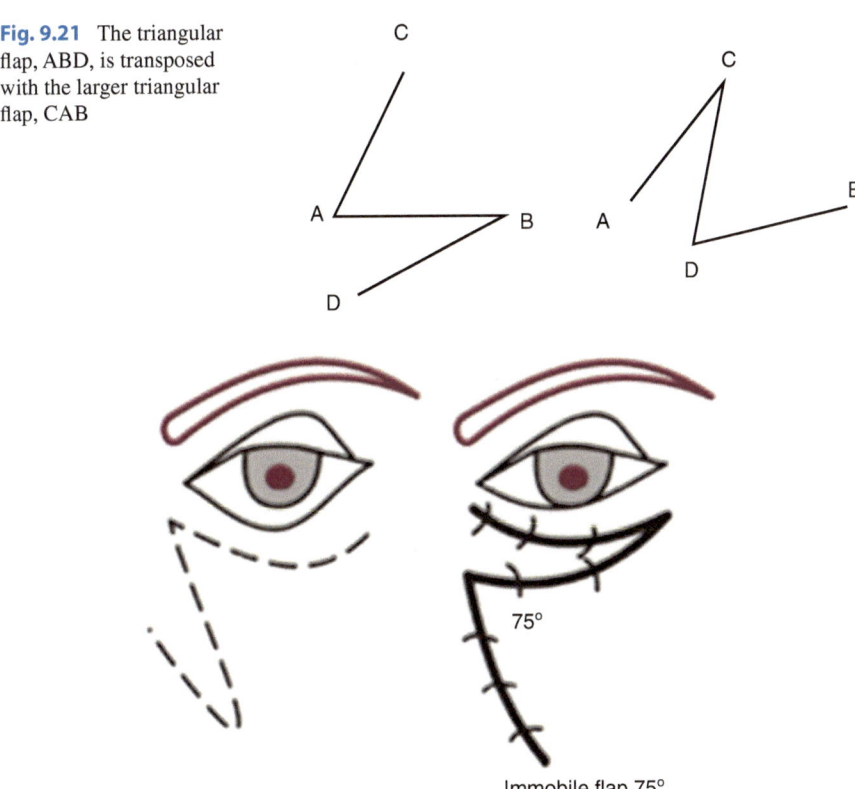

Fig. 9.21 The triangular flap, ABD, is transposed with the larger triangular flap, CAB

75°

Immobile flap 75°

Fig. 9.22 Limberg's asymmetrical Z-plasty [1]

Altering Angle Size

As previously noted, the greater the angle size, the greater the percentage increase in length. Angles greater than 60° are more difficult to transpose. This problem can be overcome by splitting the wide-angle flaps. Further modifications to the Z-plasty technique can include the four, five and six-flap Z-plasty.

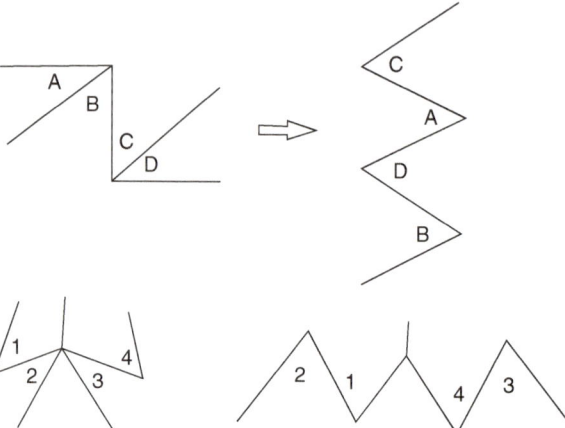

Fig. 9.23 Four and five-flap Z-plasties

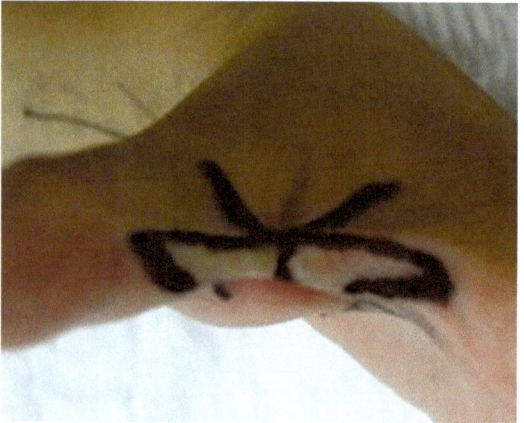

Fig. 9.24 Planning for a five-flap Z-plasty to release burn scar contracture in the first web space of a child

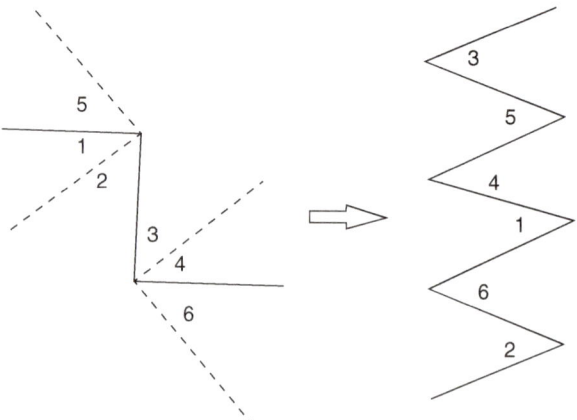

Fig. 9.25 Six-flap Z-plasty

The Jumping Man Flap

This is an extension of the five-flap Z-plasty. The V flap is made by incisions around the medial canthus and situated some distance from the baseline. It is used to correct epicanthal folds and telecanthus.

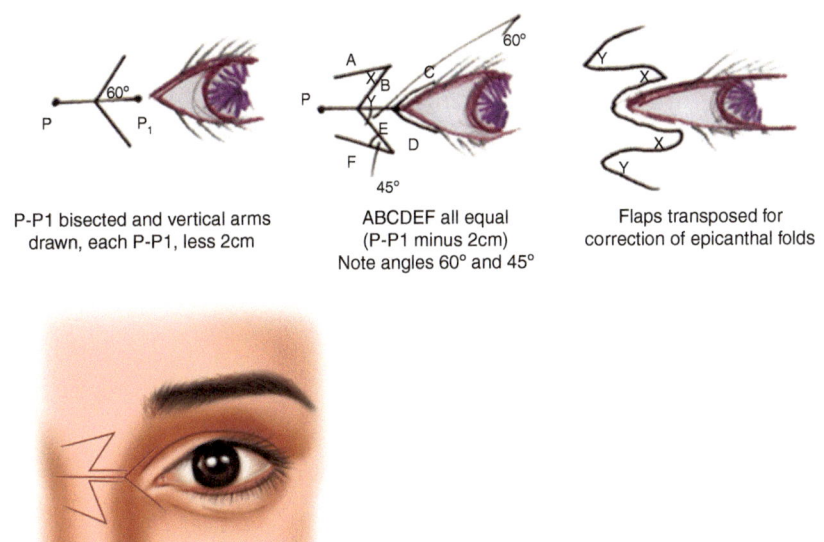

P-P1 bisected and vertical arms drawn, each P-P1, less 2cm	ABCDEF all equal (P-P1 minus 2cm) Note angles 60° and 45°	Flaps transposed for correction of epicanthal folds

Fig. 9.26 Double-opposing Z-plasties are planned with a common apex at the new site of the medial canthus. The V flap including the medial canthus is the fifth flap of this Z-plasty

Use of Z-Plasty in Flap Repairs

Following the transfer of a flap to its recipient site, there may be some distortion of the skin at the flap base. This may be simply corrected with a Z-plasty.

Similar situations using a glabellar flap or a hatchet flap can be corrected by utilizing a back-cut and converting the base of the flap to a Z-plasty. This endorses the principle of preserving as much as possible of normal skin in local flap surgery.

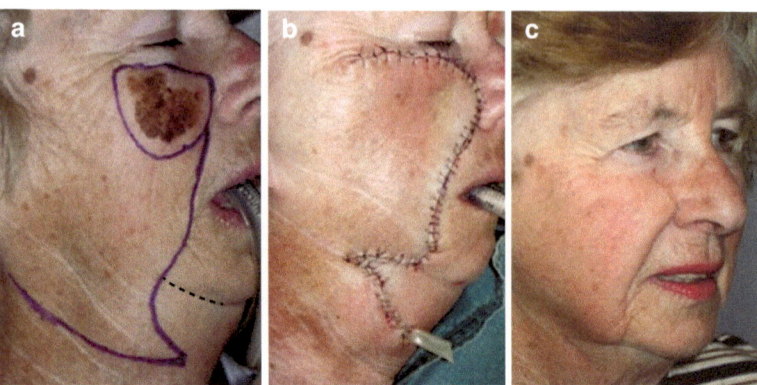

Fig. 9.27 A melanoma in-situ on the medial cheek of a 76-year-old woman (**a**), excised and repaired with a large cervico-facial rotation flap, incorpororating a Z-plasty to close the donor site (**b**). Result at 14 months (**c**) (Courtesy of Dr. Swee Tan) [8]

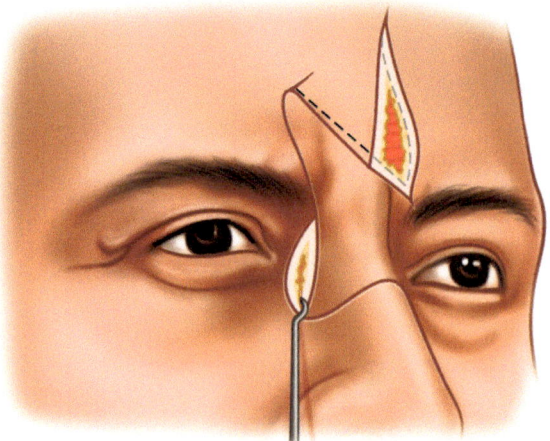

Fig. 9.28 Incorporating a Z-plasty to close the wound produced by a glabellar flap. The upper triangular part of the flap is inserted into the back-cut

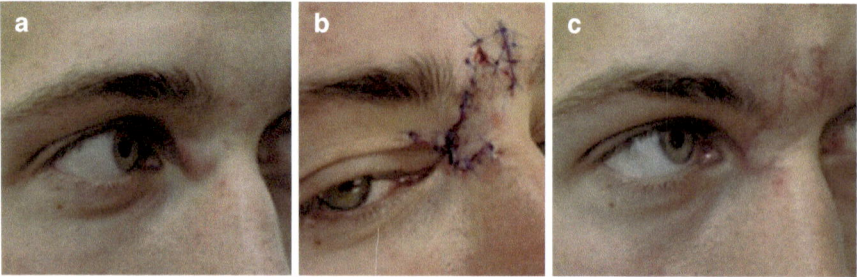

Fig. 9.29 Defect in the inner canthus following excision of a ruptured epidermoid cyst (**a**), repaired with a glabellar transposition flap incorporating a Z-plasty (**b**, **c**)

The Double Z to Rhomboid Plasty [9]

Following excision of the lesion, creating a 120°/60° rhombus, 60° Z-plasties are planned in opposite directions from the sides of the 120° angle, each limb being equal in length to the sides of the rhombus.

Four Z-plasty flaps are created, and these are transposed. The effect is to obtain half the area of required tissue from opposite sides of the defect. This procedure is versatile in that mirror image flaps can be used depending on the position and availability of lax skin.

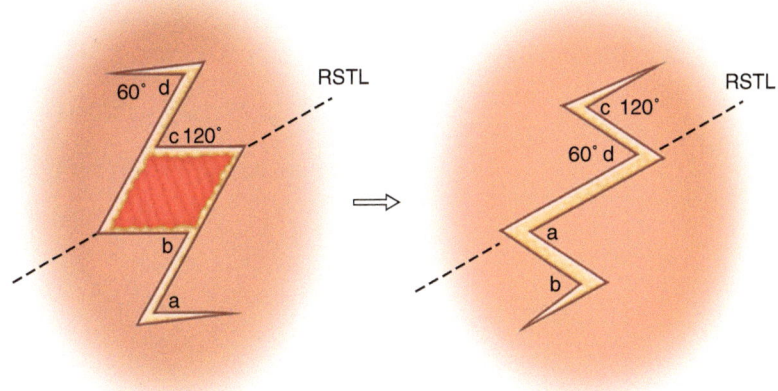

Fig. 9.30 Double-Z rhomboid plasty

Rhomboid to W-Plasty [10]

This is very similar to a double Z-plasty repair of a rhomboid defect. Opposing triangular flaps are planned and raised so that the axis of the resulting W will be in the RSTL. The triangular flaps are then transposed and advanced into the opposing triangular defect.

In general, the angle of the flap should equal that of the rhomboid and the length similar to the sidewall of the rhomboid. Both of these can be altered. With a longer flap opposite the apex of the rhomboid, the wound can be repaired as for a Z-plasty. Shorter flaps will require a V-Y advancement to complete the repair. Tissue is shared from the upper and lower parts of the triangular flaps. It is also borrowed from each side when a V-Y repair is required.

This procedure is suitable in areas where there is little spare skin for an elliptical excision and repair.

We have used this technique successfully in that area of hairless skin between the outer eyebrow and the temporal hairline.

Notes

This technique is suitable only for small skin defects. The tissue required to close the defect is provided by borrowing half the quantity from each of the two opposite sides of the defect. It is unwise to do the procedure in areas of extensive solar skin damage as the W scar may preclude further local flap surgery in that area.

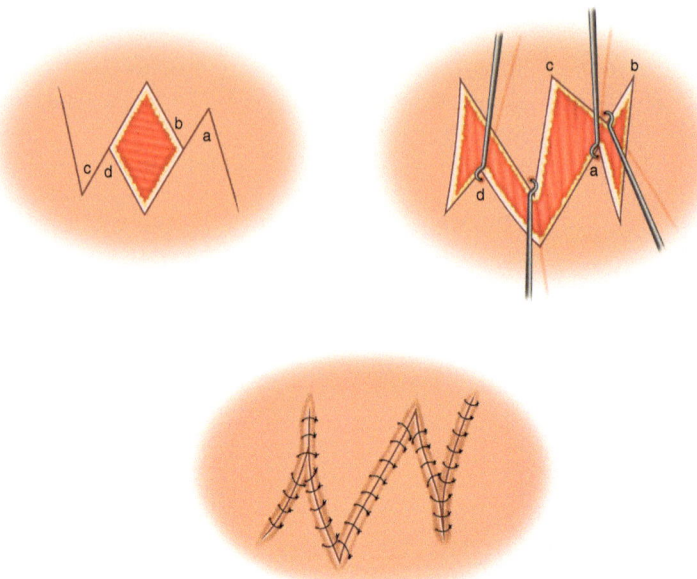

Fig. 9.31 Rhomboid to W-plasty

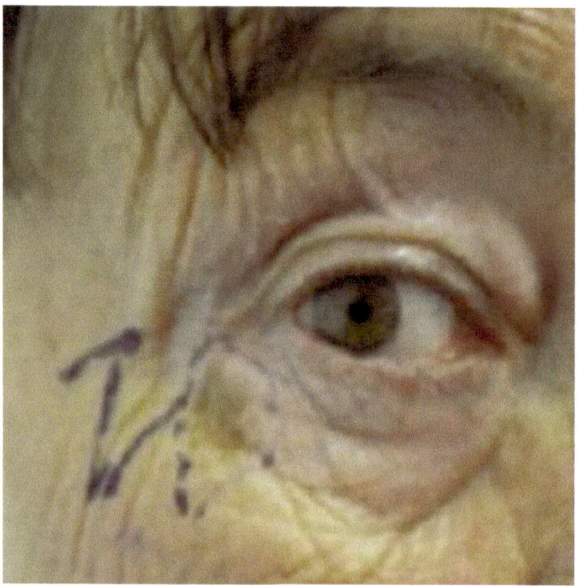

Fig. 9.32 This lesion was too big for the considered rhomboid to W-plasty in this case. See Chap. 6, Fig. 6.9 where small rotation flap chosen instead

Triangular Flaps that Advance and Interdigitate [11]

W-Plasty

This is a method of improving the appearance of scars.

Surgical method: A zigzag incision is made on each side of the scar to be treated. Small isosceles triangles are created. The flaps on each side are mobilised and advanced so that each flap interdigitates with a corresponding triangular defect.

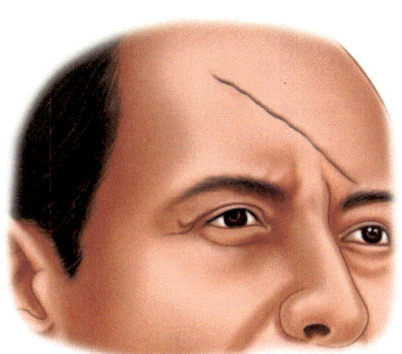

a. Oblique depressed scar of forehead

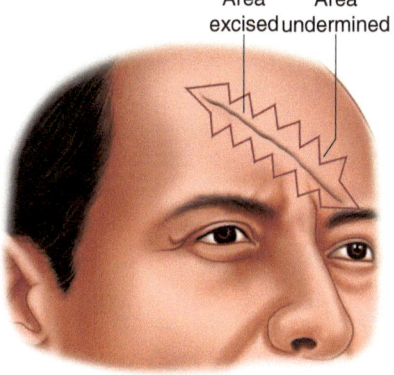

Area   Area
excised undermined

b. Pattern of multiple W-plasties

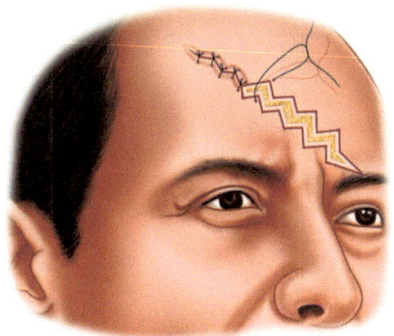

c. Interdigitation of "W" flaps

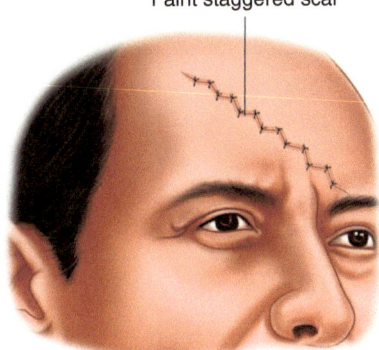

Faint staggered scar

d

Fig. 9.33 W-plasties

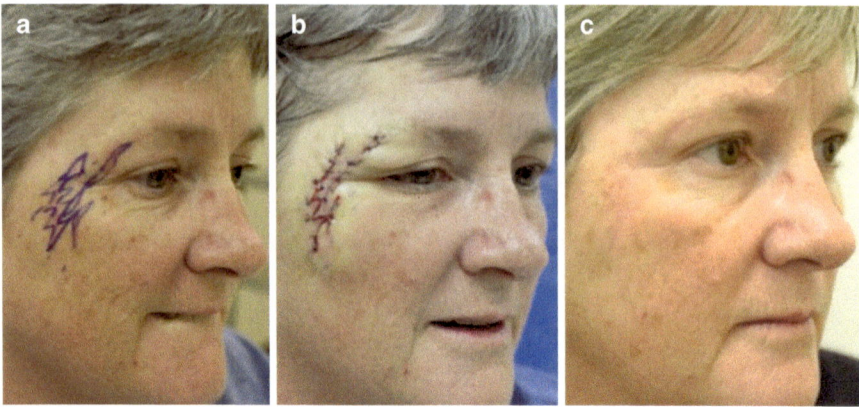

Fig. 9.34 Scar on the right periorbital/malar region of a 54-year-old woman (**a**), excised and combined with W-plasties (**b**). Result at 7 months (**c**)

The Effects of a W-Plasty

It breaks a scar into smaller components, relieving the bowstring effect of longer scars. It produces a redirection of anti-tension line scars, so that they better follow the relaxed skin tension lines. It can accomplish, by the halving technique, a situation in which the subcutaneous scar does not coincide with the zigzag cutaneous scar. This helps camouflage scars by dividing them into small segments and intermingling these segments with normal unscarred skin.

References

1. Borges AF, Gibson T (1973) The original Z-plasty. Br J Plast Surg 26(3):237–246
2. Limberg AA (1946) The planning of local plastic operations on the body surface—theory and practice (Translated by S. Anthony Wolfe 1984). Lexington, Collamore Press.
3. McGregor IA (1989) Fundamental techniques of plastic surgery and their surgical applications, 8th edn. Churchill Livingstone, Edinburgh
4. Furnas DW, Fischer GW (1971) The Z-plasty: biomechanics and mathematics. Br J Plast Surg 24(2):144–160
5. Hudson DA (2000) Some thoughts on choosing a Z-Plasty: the Z made simple. Plast Reconstr Surg 106(3):665–671
6. Brown E, Klaassen MF. Introduction to local flaps: a surgeon's handbook. 2011
7. Klaassen MF, Brown E, Behan FC. Defining local flaps: clinical applications and methods. 2016.
8. Tan ST, McKinnon CA (2006) Deep plane cervicofacial flap: a useful and versatile technique in head and neck surgery. Head Neck 28:46–55
9. Cuono CB (1983) Double z-plasty repair of large and small rhombic defects: the double-Z rhomboid. Plast Reconstr Surg 71(5):658–666
10. Strauch B, Vasconez LO, Herman CK, Lee BT (2015) Grabb's encyclopedia of flaps, 4th edn. Lippincott Williams & Wilkins, Philadelphia
11. Thomas JR, Holt GR (1989) Facial scars: incision, revision & camouflage. CV Mosby, St. Louis

Hinge Flaps

10

This is an extension of local flaps that move around a pivot point. The flap is raised on its pedicle and turned through between 90 and 180°, like the page of a book. In order to obtain more mobility, the flap can be raised on a subcutaneous pedicle, taking care to allow adequate attachment of the flap at its base to preserve blood supply.

This type of flap is useful when a structure with opposing epithelial surfaces is deficient due to trauma, neoplasm, congenital anomaly or infection. Once the lining has been restored, a further flap is required to cover the external defect.

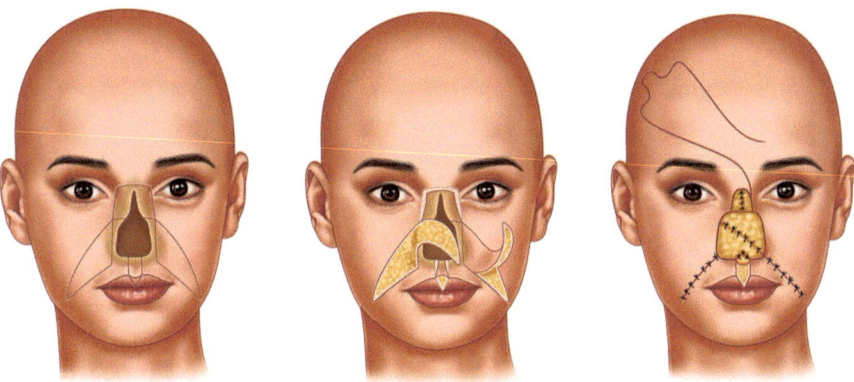

Fig. 10.1 Reconstruction of nasal lining using nasal skin and cheek skin from nasolabial folds [1, 2] based on original diagram of Joseph, 1931

© Springer International Publishing AG 2018
M.F. Klaassen et al., *Simply Local Flaps*,
https://doi.org/10.1007/978-3-319-59400-2_10

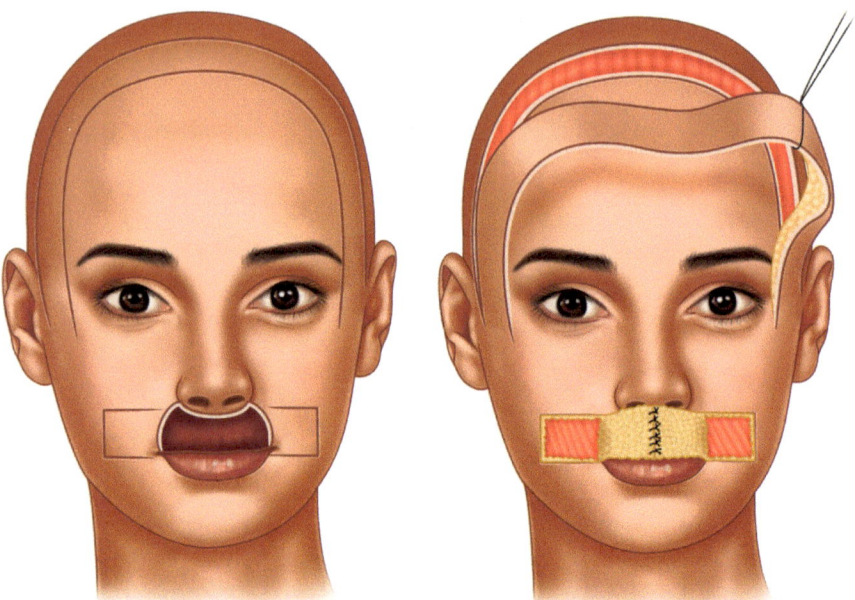

Fig. 10.2 Two cheek turnover flaps to create the inner lining in loss of the upper lip [1, 2] based on original diagram of Joseph, 1931

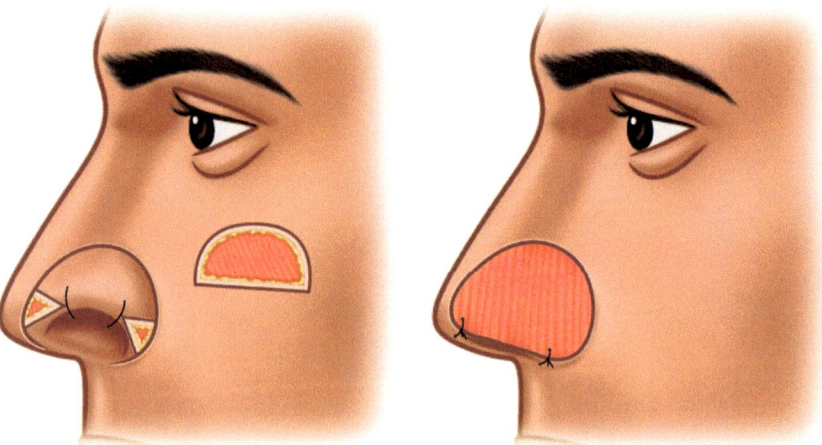

Fig. 10.3 Reconstruction of nasal lining in full thickness loss of the alar margin of the nose

The nasal lining is constructed with a turnover flap using the adjacent nasal skin. Extreme care is required in raising this flap in the vicinity of the hinge to maintain the flap's blood supply as the nasal mucosa and nasal skin are joined by scar. After setting the flap in its new position, the resulting nasal skin defect is twice the size of the original. This can now be repaired with an inferiorly based nasolabial flap.

The principle of the hinge flap has been developed further by Herbert [3].

A cheek flap is raised on a subcutaneous pedicle adjacent to the nasal defect, incorporating vascular supply around the piriform aperture. The flap is turned vertically on its hinge so that the upper and medial parts are sutured to complete reconstruction of missing nasal mucosa. The unused lower part of the flap is judiciously thinned and turned on a horizontal hinge to repair the skin defect on the nose. The flap donor site on the cheek is then repaired with a nasolabial advancement flap with a subcutaneous pedicle.

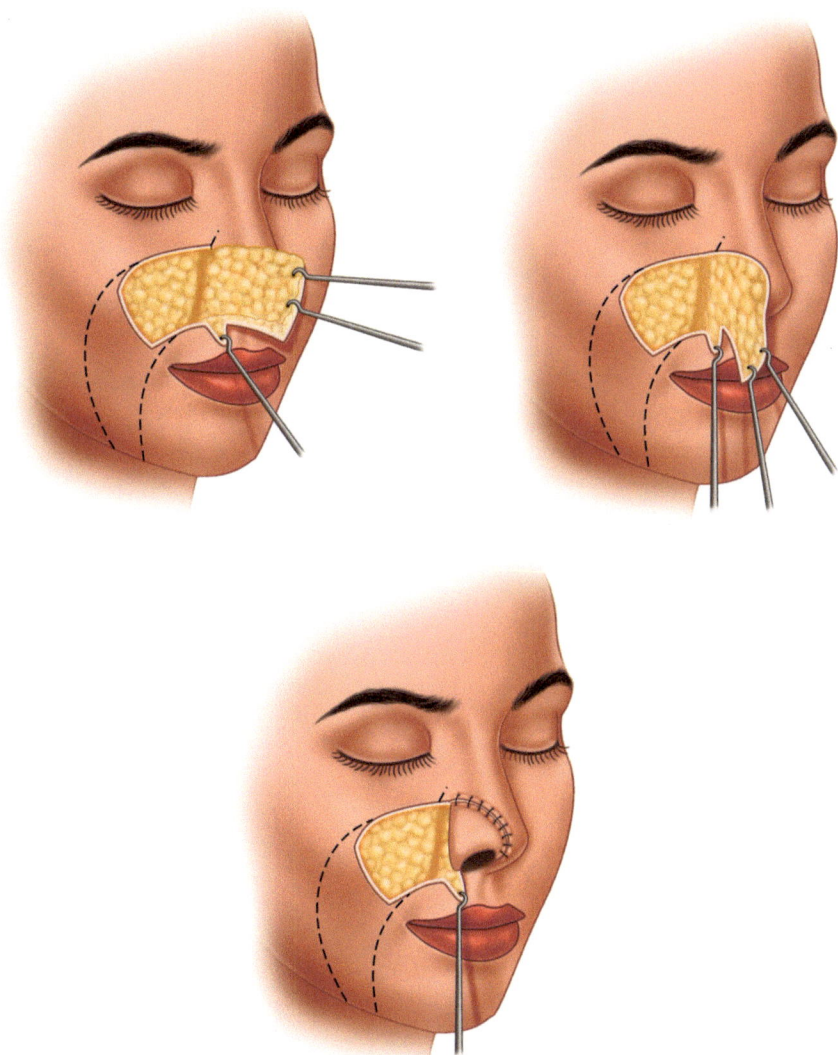

Fig. 10.4 A subcutaneous pedicle cheek advancement flap turned vertically on a hinge to provide nasal lining and the remaining portion of the flap turned horizontally to provide nasal skin cover

Classification: Hinge (single or multiple staged) flaps that move about a pivot point.

Clinical scenario I: Heminose reconstruction in a 35-year-old man post-extended hemimaxillectomy/hemi-rhinectomy for sarcoma of the right maxilla. The large orbito-rhino-maxillary defect had been originally reconstructed with latissimus dorsi myocutaneous free flap for large orbito-rhino-maxillary defect, followed by post-operative adjuvant radiotherapy. The patient was ready for staged heminose reconstruction with lining, support and cover 1 year later.

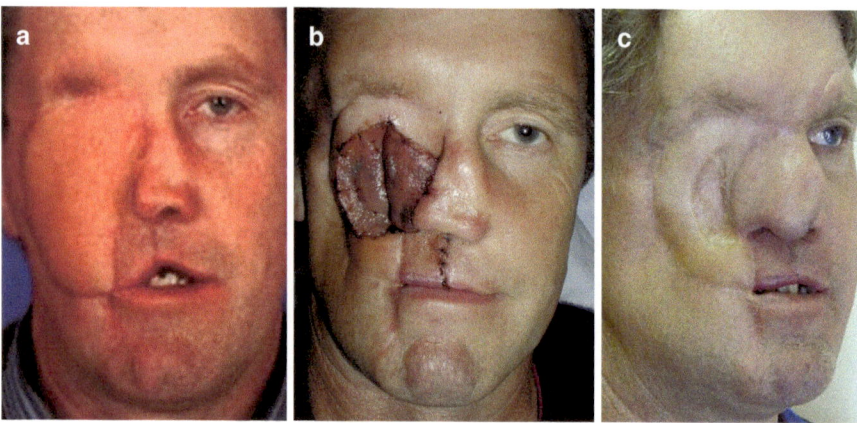

Fig. 10.5 35-year-old man with a latissimus dorsi myocutaneous free flap repair, following radical surgery for sarcoma of the right maxilla (**a**). The hinge flap was performed (**b**) and further staged reconstruction using a forehead flap (**c**)

Clinical scenario II: Melanoma in-situ confirmed on excision biopsy of a changing pigmented lesion on the plantar aspect of the left second toe of a 29-year-old woman. Wider excision was performed, and the plantar toe defect was repaired with a staged cross toe flap, hinged from the dorsal surface and medial aspect of the left third toe and a full thickness skin graft to the donor site as well as the exposed pedicle.

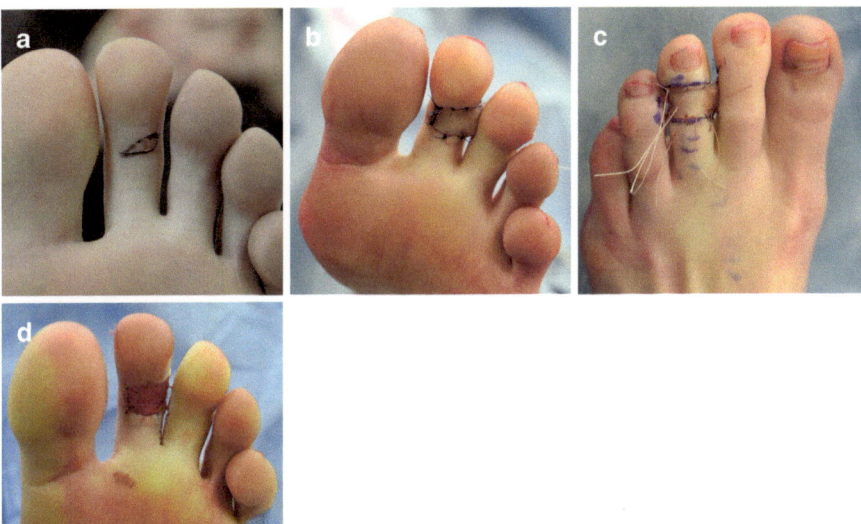

Fig. 10.6 A melanoma in-situ on the plantar aspect of the left second toe of a 32-year-old woman (**a**), widely excised and repaired with a cross toe flap from the dorsal third toe (**b**, **c**). Result 2 weeks following division of the flap (**d**)

Cross Finger Flap

This is similar to Fig. 10.6 above and applied in the hand for repairs to cover partial pulp amputations, exposed flexor tendons in the fingers and for the correction of chronic finger flexion contractures following burn injuries [4, 5].

The cross finger flap is divided at 2 weeks. The thenar flap is another example of using the Hinge principle in Hand Surgery.

The hinge flap can be used in other situations such as reconstructing the urethra in patients with hypospadias.

A similar technique can be used to provide muscle padding in repair of pressure areas and subcutaneous tissue to augment depressed scars.

References

1. Joseph J. Rhinoplasty and facial plastic surgery with a supplement on mammaplasty, An atlas and textbook by Prof Dr. J. Joseph of Berlin English translation by Stanley Milstein B.A., M.A., M.D. (1987) Columella Press/Phoenix. 1931.
2. Olivari N (2008) Practical plastic and reconstructive surgery. An atlas of operations and techniques. Kaden, Heidelberg
3. Herbert DC, De Geus JJ (1975) Nasolabial subcutaneous pedicle flaps. Br J Plast Surg 28:90
4. Jackson IT, Brown GE (1970) A method of treating chronic flexion contractures of the fingers. Br J Plast Surg 23:373–379
5. Kappel DA, Burech JG (1985) The cross-finger flap; an established reconstructive procedure. Hand Clin 1:677–683
6. Herbert DC (1979) A subcutaneous pedicled cheek flap for reconstruction of alar defects. Br J Plast Surg 31:79–92

Recommended Traditional Local Flaps

11

Rotation Scalp Flap

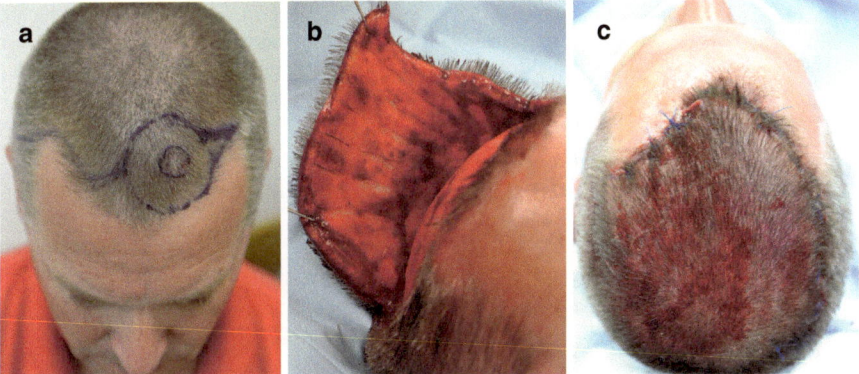

Fig. 11.1 A nodular malignant melanoma on the frontal scalp in a 50-year-old man (**a**), widely excised and repaired with a large rotation scalp flap with galeal scoring (**b**), achieving closure of the left frontal defect (**c**)

© Springer International Publishing AG 2018
M.F. Klaassen et al., *Simply Local Flaps*,
https://doi.org/10.1007/978-3-319-59400-2_11

Paramedian Forehead Flap

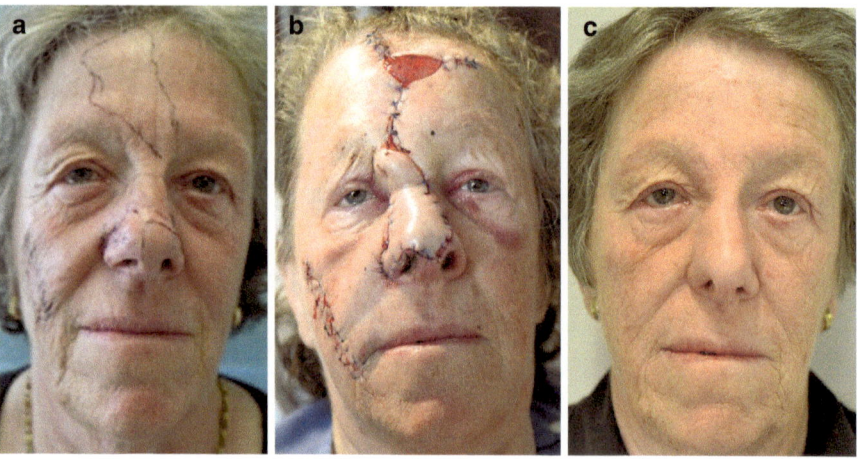

Fig. 11.2 A recurrent BCC on the nose of a 65-year-old woman (**a**), excised and repaired with a left paramedian forehead interpolated flap (**b**). The forehead donor site was partially closed with sliding flaps and the residual wound left to heal by secondary intention. Result at 5 months (**c**)

Biwinged Excision/Sliding Advancement Flaps

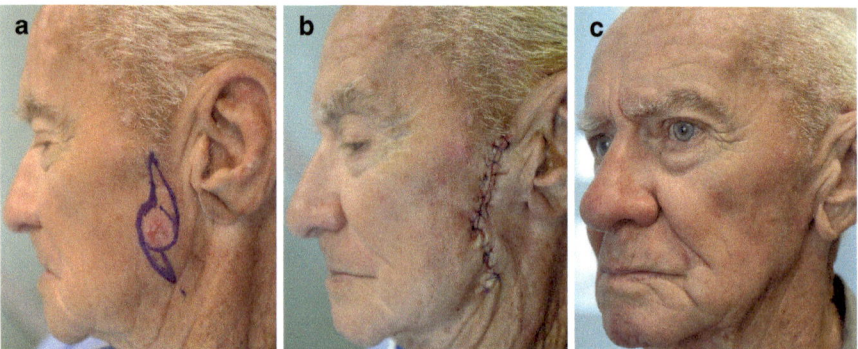

Fig. 11.3 A moderately differentiated infiltrating SCC on the left cheek area in an 87-year-old man (**a**), widely excised and repaired with biwinged sliding advancement local flaps (**b**). Result at 6 weeks (**c**). A good alternative in this situation would be a double hatchet flap

Sigmoid Oblique Advancement Flap [1]

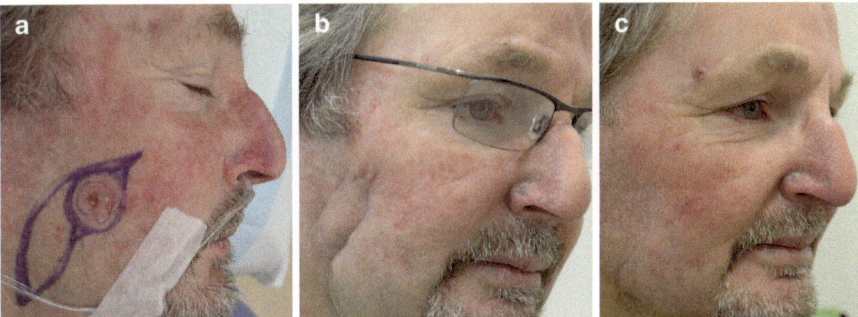

Fig. 11.4 An infiltrating BCC on the right lateral cheek of a 58-year-old man (**a**), widely excised and repaired with a sigmoid oblique advancement flap. Result at 3 months (**b**) and 12 months (**c**). Note a new BCC on the right temple and previous forehead rhinoplasty

Nasolabial Flap (Superiorly Based)

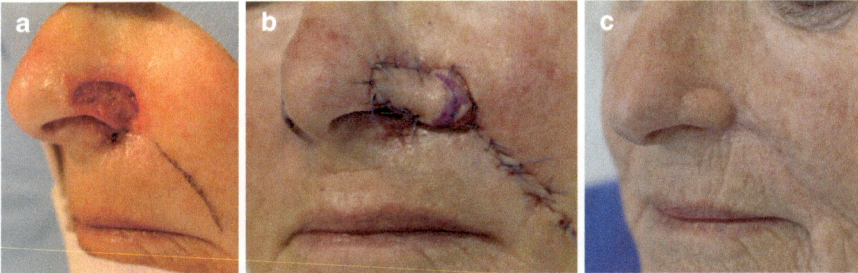

Fig. 11.5 Two-stage nasolabial interpolated flap was used for defect of left alar region of the nose, following margin-controlled wide excision of infiltrating BCC for a 73-year-old woman (**a**, **b**). Result at 6 months (**c**)

Dorsal Nasoaxial Flap

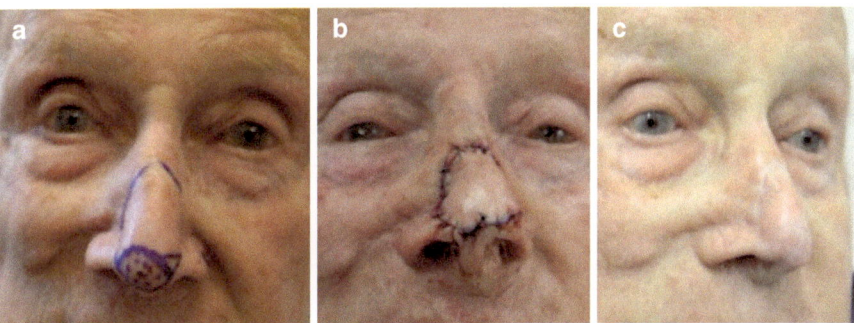

Fig. 11.6 A nodular BCC at the tip of the nose in a 92-year-old man (**a**), excised and reconstructed with a short dorsal nasoaxial flap (**b**). Result at 18 months (**c**)

Glabellar Flap

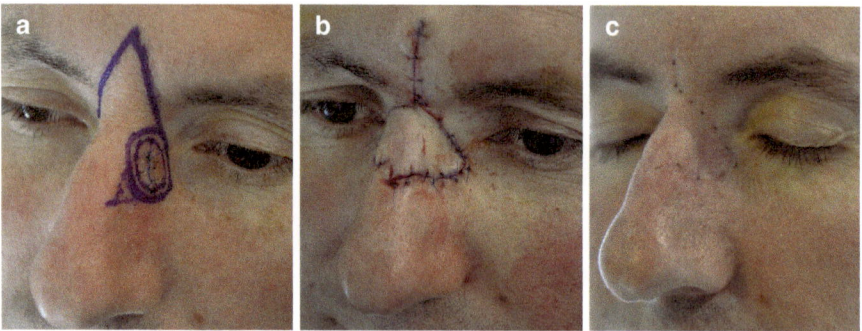

Fig. 11.7 A biopsy-proven infiltrating BCC of the left side of the nose/medial canthal region, in a 45-year-old man (**a**), excised and repaired with a glabellar transposition flap (**b**). Result at 3 years with marking pen outlining the original flap (**c**)

Transposition Cheek Flap

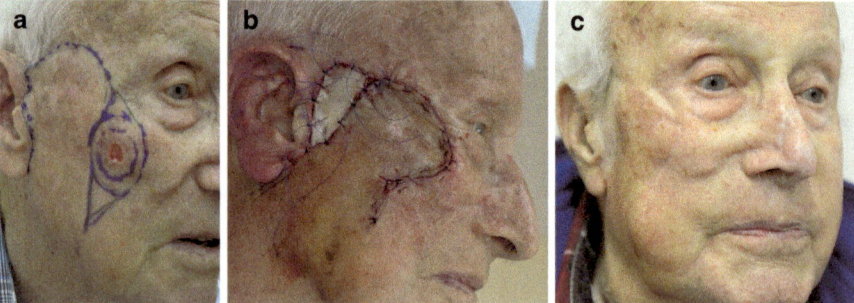

Fig. 11.8 An ulcerated infiltrating BCC on the right cheek of a 91-year-old man (**a**), excised and repaired with an inferiorly based lateral cheek transposition flap (**b**). Due to previous surgery on the cheek, there was inadequate skin to repair the donor site, which was repaired with a postauricular full thickness skin graft (**b**). Result at 2 years (**c**)

Karapandzic Flaps [2]

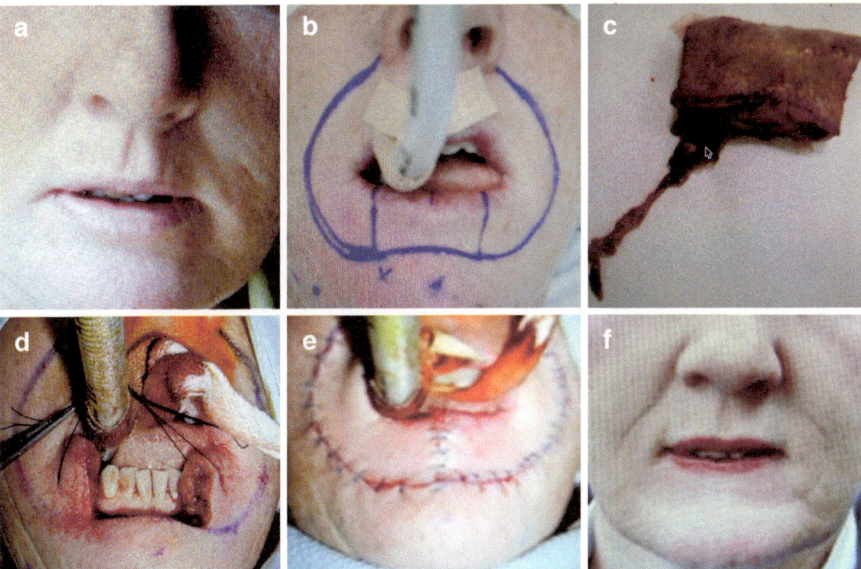

Fig. 11.9 A desmoplastic malignant melanoma on the central lower lip in a young woman (**a**), requiring a wide full thickness excision of the lower lip including the right mental nerve (**b–d**). Bilateral Karapandzic flaps were used to reconstruct the lower lip defect (**e**), followed by post-operative adjuvant radiotherapy. Result at 12 months (**f**)

Dorsal Hand Flap [3]

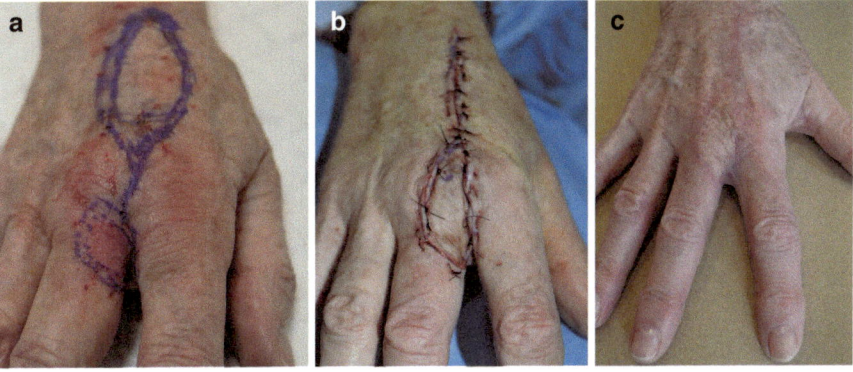

Fig. 11.10 A biopsy-proven SCC in-situ on the radial aspect of the proximal phalanx of the middle finger/webspace of the right hand, of a 74-year-old woman (**a**). The lesion was excised, and the defect was repaired with a dorsal hand propeller flap (**b**). The result at 8 weeks (**c**)

References

1. Ono I, Gunji H, Sato M, Kaneko F (1993) Use of the oblique island flap in excision of small facial tumours. Plast Reconstr Surg 91(7):1245–1251
2. Karapandzic M (1974) Reconstruction of lip defects by local arterial flaps. Br J Plast Surg 27(1):93–97
3. Quaba AA, Davison PM (1990) The distally-based dorsal hand flap. Br J Plast Surg 43:28–39

Part III

Modern Local Flaps

Chapter 12: Keystone Flap Concepts

The perforator island local flap concepts of Assoc. Prof. Felix Behan who has pioneered the keystone flap will be summarized.

Chapter 13: Favoured Keystone Flap Applications

The ten best clinical cases to illustrate the lead author's use of the keystone local flap concept will be presented.

Chapter 14: Combination Flaps

For certain defects, especially involving the face, a combination of local flaps is the best option.

Keystone Flap Concepts

12

Anatomy and Physiology

Historically Behan and Wilson [1] began researching this concept whilst based in London in 1973. The *angiotome* concept, which is the key anatomical/physiological basis for this island perforator local fasciocutaneous *advancement* flap, defines an area of the skin that survives when cut as a flap, supplied by an axial vessel extended by its communication with branches from the adjacent vessel. The concept emphasises the role of the dermatome and the intrinsic neurocutaneous vascular supply of the human skin. This is essential to the planning of bespoke keystone perforator island flaps (KPIFs).

The fasciocutaneous island flaps that Behan was using to cover compound lower limb fractures in the 1990s developed into the keystone perforator island flaps. Serendipitously he combined the dermatome pattern of design with the concept of angiotome vascular perfusion [2].

Essentially a dermatome associated with somite development is an area of the skin supplied by a spinal nerve. If a spinal nerve is to develop from the notochord (primitive streak area), it must have an arteriovenous support network for this autonomic-somatic neural complex. The basic embryological principle is confirmed. The neurovascular structures subsequently become arborized, which account for their distal perfusion from minute vascular links.

Lymphatic development must also accompany such arborisation with development and growth. This simple aide-memoire of a dermatomal link, based on a fascial support without skeletonizing the perforator source, allows the accompanying lymphatic and autonomic fibres to be retained.

Finally, there are humoural factors (nitrous oxide), which also operate within this scheme.

The keystone perforator island flaps are robust and complications infrequent—except when there is wound dehiscence from premature removal of sutures. Wound closure under tension is the norm.

© Springer International Publishing AG 2018
M.F. Klaassen et al., *Simply Local Flaps*,
https://doi.org/10.1007/978-3-319-59400-2_12

The KIPFs are based on arterial perforators, their venae comitantes and the fine vascular networks that accompany nerves. Recent research into the origin of stem cells from the primitive spinal cord suggests that regularity pathways of stem cells and angiogenesis play a collaborative role in sustaining vascularity in the healing of these flaps. The stem cells are the ancestor cells, which self-renew and produce a variety of mature functioning cells in all tissues. Stem cell self-renewal is an ability controlled by intrinsic genetic pathways, as well as being influenced by extrinsic signals from the stem cell microenvironment.

Minor indirect cutaneous vessels are the main perforators for keystone flaps, and vessels accompany the nerves—these are key principles underpinning the angiotome concept of the keystone perforator island local fasciocutaneous flap.

The term 'keystone' refers to the way the flap locks into the defect employing a double V-Y advancement. Physiology plays an important role in the predictability and safety of these flaps—there is a complex interplay of denervation of the autonomic and somatic afferent nervous systems after raising the flaps. Behan calls this the immediate vascular augmentation concept (IVAC) [3].

It is proper and relevant to mention that the keystone flap has elements of the traditional flaps. In fact it is a logical extension of the traditional flap principles being an advancement flap, based on an island of subcutaneous tissue through which course the important perforator vessels. The skin and subcutaneous tissue adjacent to the ellipse on the opposite side to the keystone flap, also advance to complete wound closure. Some undermining and sliding flap element may be required, but not usually. The double V-Y closure of the keystone flap donor site is also a traditional method.

Flap Design

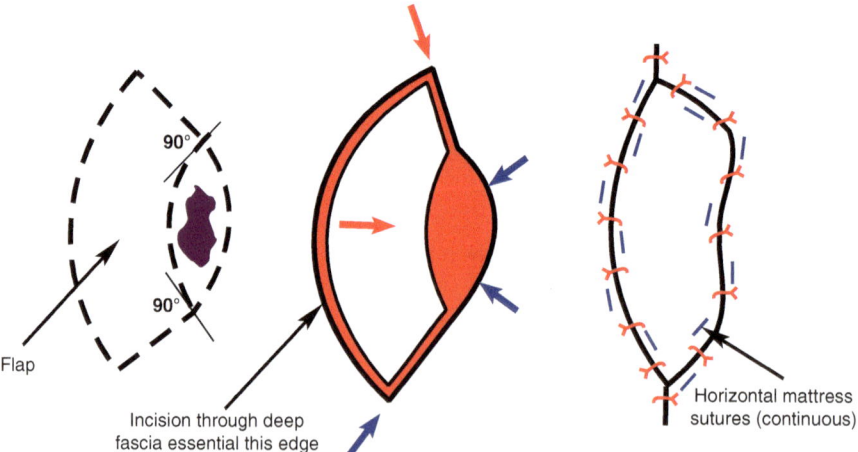

Fig. 12.1 Keystone flap design concept (Behan) [5]

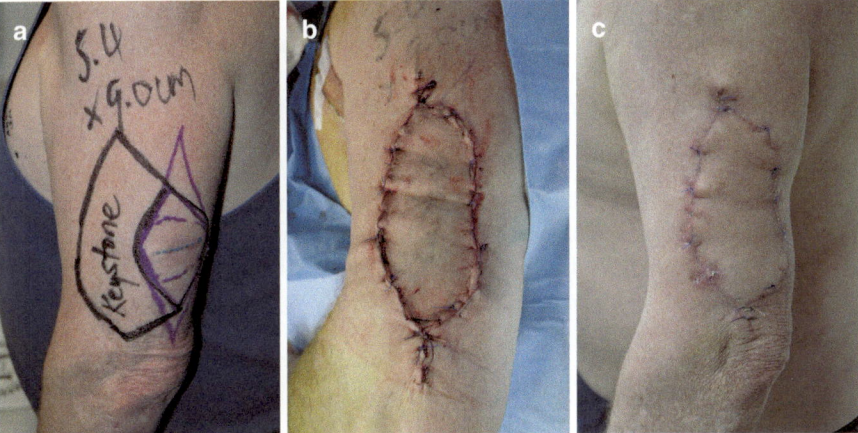

Fig. 12.2 A thick nodular melanoma on the left lateral arm of a 63-year-old man, underwent a wide excision (**a**). The excisional defect measured 9.0 × 5.4 cm and was repaired with a keystone flap (**b**). Result at 3 weeks (**c**)

The standard and simplest design of the keystone flap is based on a fusiform or elliptical excision of the lesion or wound (Fig. 12.1). A curved trapezoid-shaped flap with the shortest side being contiguous with one side of the defect to be repaired is designed. The longitudinal axis of the flap should run in the lines of the dermatome of the skin area. Flaps should be planned over muscle bellies where possible, to improve perforator capture.

Technically, the complete release of the deep fascia overlying biceps and brachialis in Fig. 12.2 was very important. This allowed stretching and movement of the feeding perforating vessels into the flap as it is doubly advanced from the superior and inferior vectors. There is also some advancement of the posterior wound edge.

Surgical Technique for Keystone Flap

The release of the deep fascia is the significant surgical technique that took me some time to fully appreciate.

The keystone design is straightforward. The flap should follow the axis of the dermatomal lines and be centred over well-vascularized muscle bellies.

Draw a line around the edge of the tumour, select the appropriate excision margin and mark this as an outer circle around the tumour edge. Convert the circular cut out into a short fusiform or ellipse (the kind that will give you dog-ears at either end), and then draw from the apex of each half ellipse a line at 90° to the apex. Connect these two oblique lines with an arc, and the width of the keystone flap should be at least the width of the excision defect. I always make it 10–20% larger. The long arc of the flap, away from the excision edge of the defect, is incised through the skin, subcutaneous tissue and then the deep fascia. Avoid damaging any vessels or nerves that may be in the path of this incision. The oblique lines are incised into the subcutaneous tissue with preservation of all venous drainage vessels. The deep fascia is not divided in the oblique line incisions, but if necessary it can be divided and the veins are preserved.

The best instrument for advancing the keystone flap towards the defect is a skin hook. Blunt dissection with fine scissors will help release any tethering fascial fibres. Tack the flap into place with either 3/0 or 2/0 Prolene on the trunk and limbs. For the face I would use 5/0 or 4/0 Prolene. The Lorryman or double-hitch suture of Attwood is excellent for initial tacking. The lateral leading edges of the keystone flap often need trimming to fit neatly into the defect. Complete the flap repair with a running horizontal mattress suture. *Never ever use any deep sutures*— these have the potential to strangulate the perforating vessels, which are the blood supply.

The back corners of the keystone flap donor site are closed as for a V-Y repair (Fig. 12.2).

For small, moderate or very large keystone flaps, the surgical dissection planes and release of the deep fascia to facilitate mobilization are the same.

Variants of the keystone flap design include direct closure of the secondary defect (as in Fig. 12.2), skin grafting of the secondary defect, double opposing keystone flaps (Yin Yang variant) and the closing keystone (Omega variant). In the Omega variant, the central third of the flap remains anchored to the island pedicle, and each outer third is undermined at a subcutaneous plane and transposed to make good the defect (see Figs. 13.14 and 13.17). Sometimes small split skin grafts are required for the secondary defects of the Omega variant. The various designs and applications of the keystone flap are illustrated in Chap. 13.

The keystone perforator island local flap has become the preferred option for the lead author in his surgical practice. The many advantages include it's simplicity, design variability, robustness and reliability in young healthy patients and older patients with co-morbidities. It is quick and efficient, and the reduced operating time is a real bonus for the less robust patient. Most cases are easily performed under local anaesthetic. The post-operative pain is minimal and the procedure well tolerated by all patients. The aesthetic reconstructive results are also very satisfactory from head to foot and all regions of the body [5].

References

1. Behan FC (1992) The fasciocutaneous island flap: an extension of the angiotome concept. Aust NZ J Surg 62(11):874–886
2. Behan FC (1994) Fasciocutaneous island flaps for orthopaedic management in lower limb—reconstruction using dermatomal precincts. Aust NZ J Surg 64:155–166
3. Behan FC, Findlay M, Lo CH (2012) The keystone perforator island flap concept. Churchill Livingstone, Sydney
4. Behan FC, Findlay M, Lo CH (2016) The keystone perforator flap in the management of malignant melanoma. Elsevier Australia, Chatswood
5. Klaassen M.F., Brown E. and Behan F.C. (2016), Defining local flaps: clinical applications and methods

Favoured Keystone Flap Applications

13

Cheek

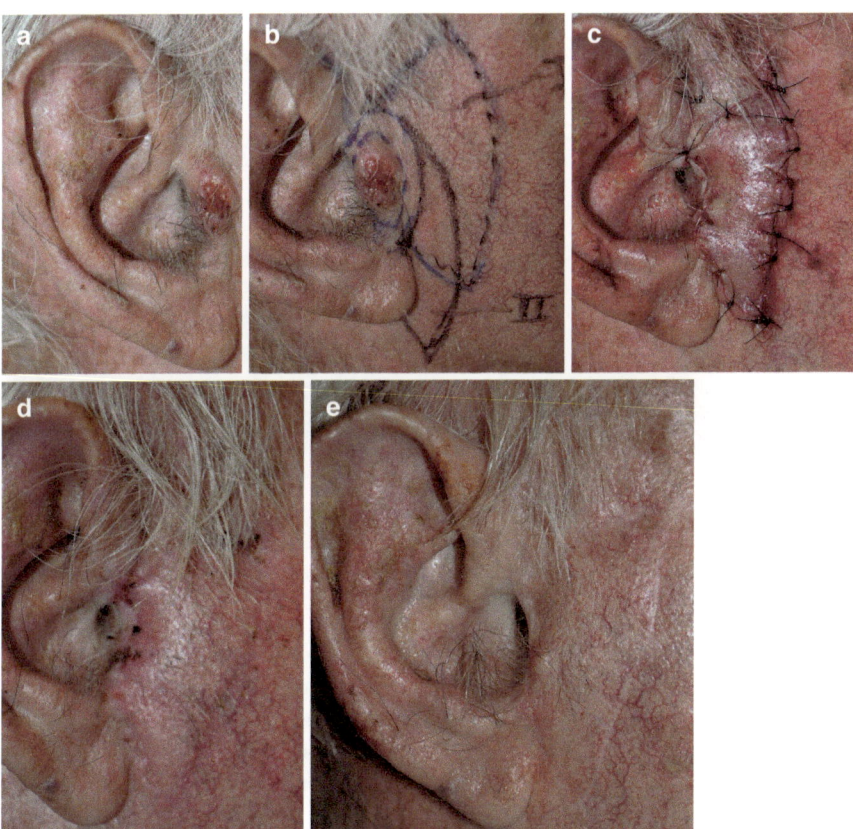

Fig. 13.1 A 74-year-old man with an ulcerated BCC involving the tragus of his right ear (**a**). My repair options included a sigmoid oblique advancement flap or my first keystone flap (**b**). The keystone was chosen with the results immediately (**c**), 1 month (**d**) and 18 months (**e**)

© Springer International Publishing AG 2018
M.F. Klaassen et al., *Simply Local Flaps*,
https://doi.org/10.1007/978-3-319-59400-2_13

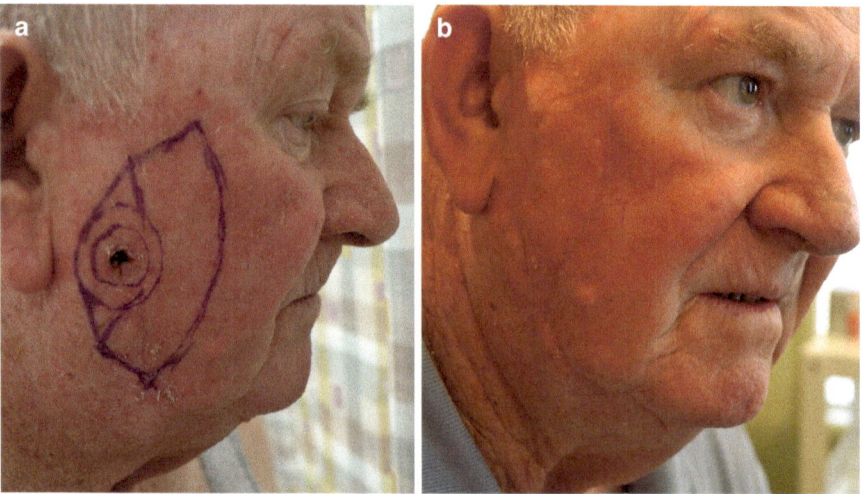

Fig. 13.2 A large preauricular BCC on the right cheek widely excised and repaired with a keystone flap (**a**). Result at 3 months (**b**)

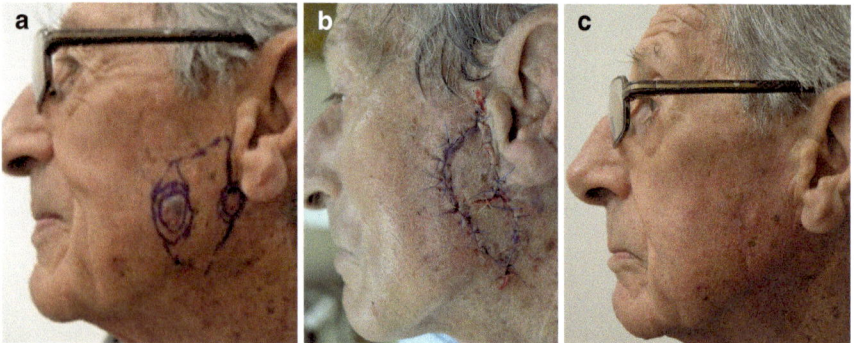

Fig. 13.3 A 90-year-old man with two cheek BCCs on the lateral cheek (**a**). A keystone flap was planned between the two excisions and double advancement superiorly and inferiorly enabled repair (**b**). A central dog-ear was excised without risk to flap vascularity. The result at 4 months (**c**)

Notes

There are many alternative local flaps that could have been applied in these cases.

Keystone flaps can be designed for the cheek and lateral face with the flap margins following the RSTLs. This helps achieve more aesthetic reconstructions. These flaps heal rapidly because of their excellent blood supply; trapdoor scarring is rare and post-operative discomfort is minimal.

Lateral Nose

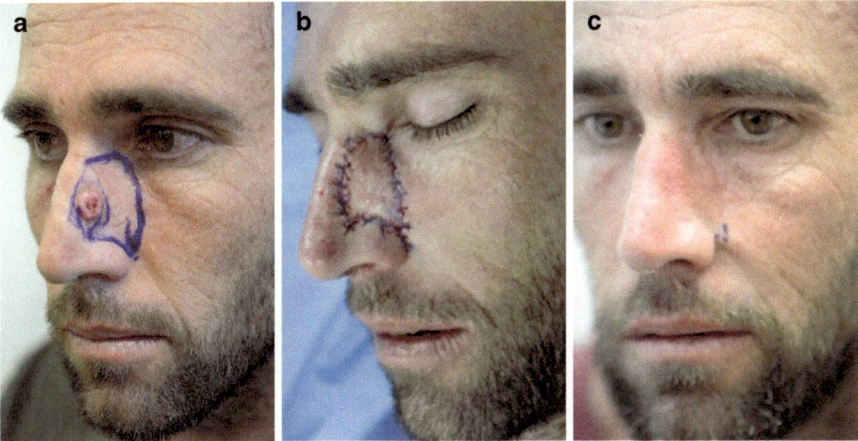

Fig. 13.4 A rapidly growing SCC on the left lateral nose of a 35-year-old man (**a**). Wide excision was performed down to cartilage and reconstruction with a keystone perforator island local flap (**b**). Result at 3 years (**c**)

Upper Lip

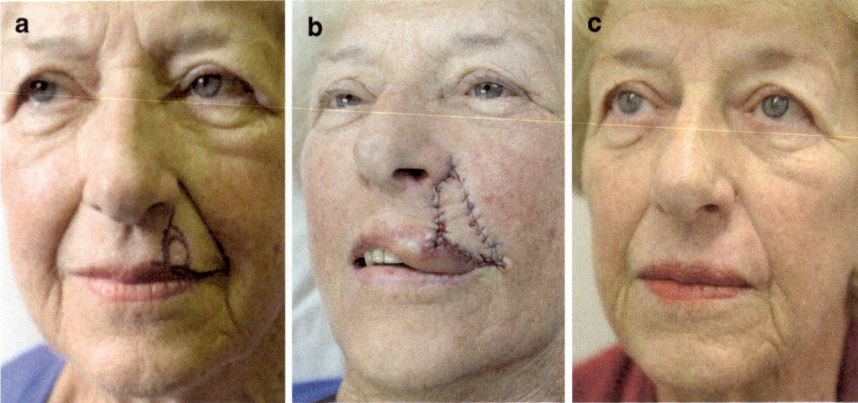

Fig. 13.5 An atypical actinic keratosis on this 73-year-old woman's left upper lip (**a**) was excised and repaired with keystone flap (**b**). Result at 4 months (**c**)

Notes

The keystone flaps in the two cases illustrated have allowed camouflage of the final scars in the aesthetic subunits of the lateral nose and lateral upper lip/nasolabial zone as well as avoiding distortion of key anatomical landmarks: the nasal tip, alar base, philtral column and Cupid's bow.

Forehead, Temple and Scalp

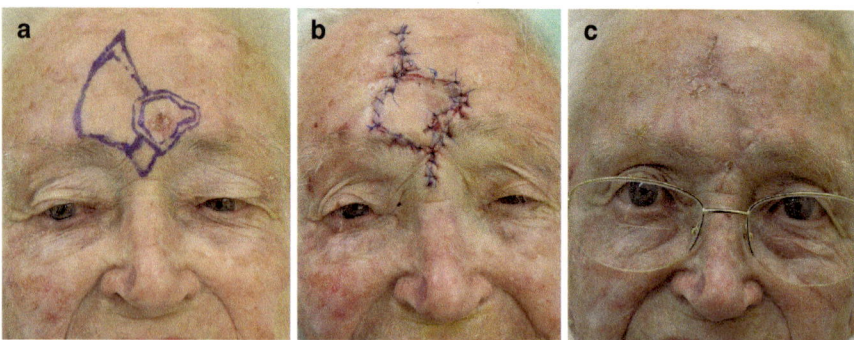

Fig. 13.6 A recurrent BCC within a skin graft in the glabellar region (**a**) was excised and repaired with a bespoke keystone flap (**b**). The keystone flap shape was modified to accommodate the shape of the defect, using an Omega design. Result at 3 weeks (**c**)

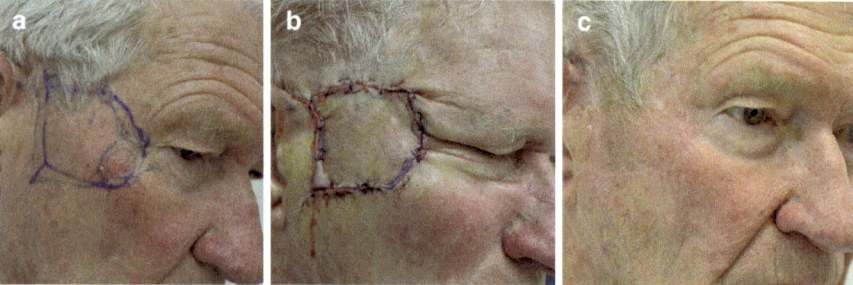

Fig. 13.7 A BCC right temple/malar junction in a 79-year-old man was excised, and the defect was repaired with a keystone flap designed to match the RSTLs (**a**). Results immediate (**b**) and nearly 4 years post-operatively (**c**). An alternative option would have been a cheek rotation flap

Notes

The glabellar region has significant laxity and spare skin, which lends itself to keystone local flap design.

Like the traditional local flaps, the keystone local flaps can be variable and flexible in design, to suit the particular surgical defect or problem. Our clinical experience has been that they are surprisingly painless in the early post-operative period.

The sympathectomy effect and the denervation of the flap and neighbouring skin are a theory that has been argued.

The double advancement of the keystone perforator island flap design is inherent in the converging vectors of advancement, obliquely towards the wound. The far side of the wound also advances naturally towards the advancing keystone flap. Although the skin closure may initially appear to be under tension, there is in fact no tension at the deeper level. This is due to the release of the deep fascia. Deep sutures are avoided as they could potentially strangulate the vital perforating vessels, advancing within the mobile island of subcutaneous tissue.

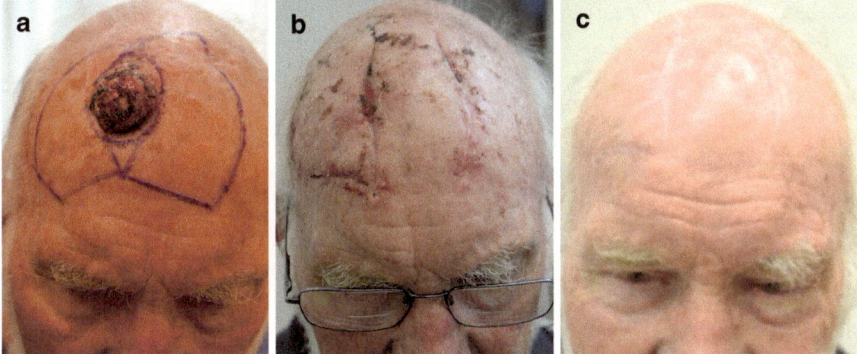

Fig. 13.8 Double keystone flaps used to close the frontal scalp defect following excision of an ulcerated SCC in an 86-year-old man (**a**). Early (**b**) and 9 month post-operative results (**c**)

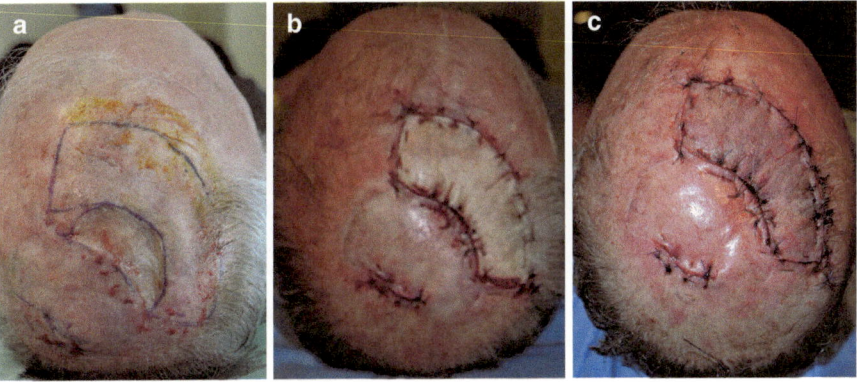

Fig. 13.9 A 67-year-old man, unhappy with the skin-grafted secondary defect on his scalp following previous skin cancer excision and rotation flap repair (**a**). The grafted area was excised and repaired with a keystone flap. Results immediately (**b**) and 24 hours post-operatively (**c**)

Notes

Keystone flaps on the scalp can be difficult and may in some instances require two flaps. A key principle for scalp keystone flaps is to retain the bipedicled galeal attachments for venous drainage. The only keystone flap I have lost with necrosis was one of two flaps for a woman on anticoagulants, whose post-operative scalp flap bleeding caused a venous outflow obstruction (see Chap. 17 on *Complications & How to Manage*).

Smaller keystone flaps for scalp defects move incredibly well to provide tension free closure. The initial blanching in the flap can be a concern, and I always check the flap vascularity at 24 hours after surgery to allay my fears of ischaemia!

For larger scalp defects, traditional classic rotation or transposition local flaps, with or without skin grafts, are recommended.

Neck

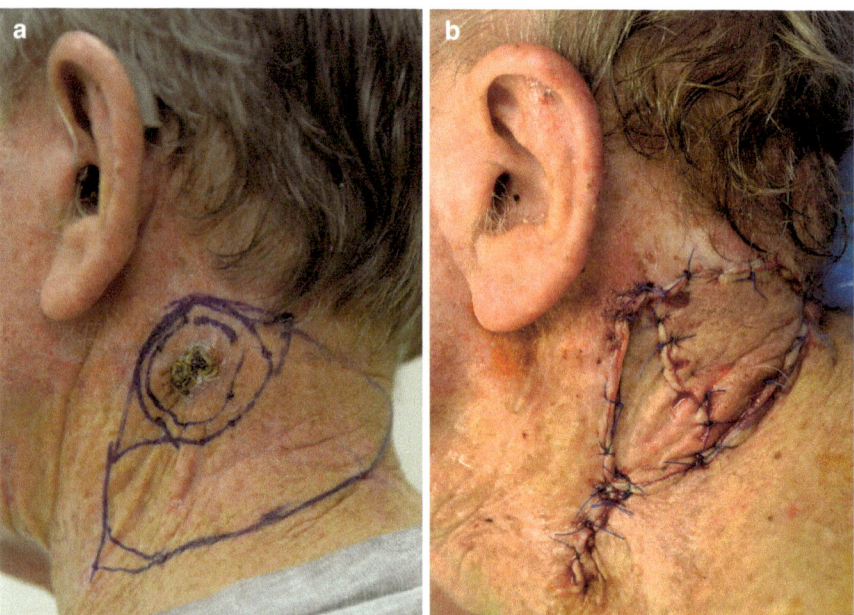

Fig. 13.10 Wide excision of an ulcerated SCC on the left posterior triangle of neck in a 55-year-old man (**a**) excised and repaired with keystone flap using the Omega variant (**b**)

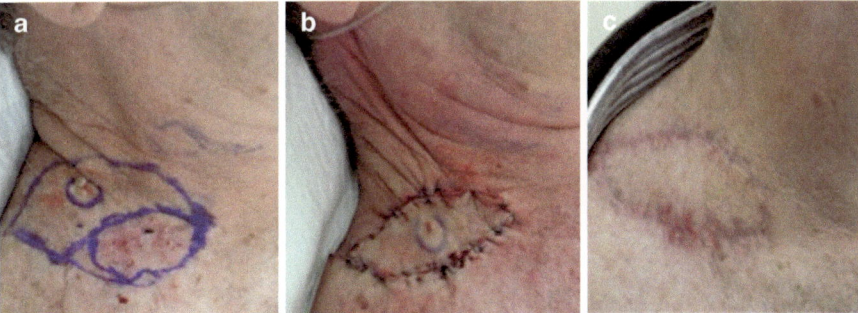

Fig. 13.11 A multifocal BCC right anterior neck (**a**) excised and repaired with a keystone flap in a 62-year-old man. Immediate (**b**) and 6 week post-operative results (**c**)

Shoulder

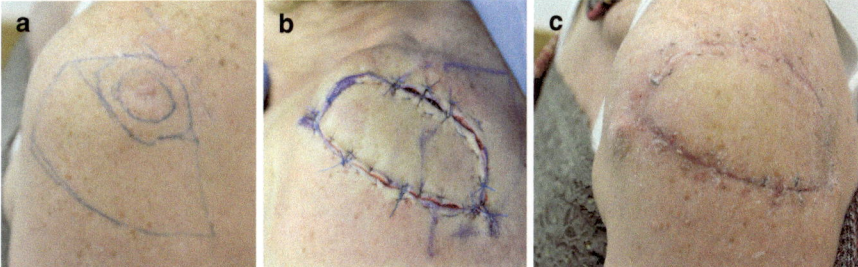

Fig. 13.12 Classical keystone flap used to repair a large defect on left deltoid region of a 75-year-old woman following wide excision of recurrent BCC (**a**). Immediate (**b**) and 1 month post-operative results (**c**)

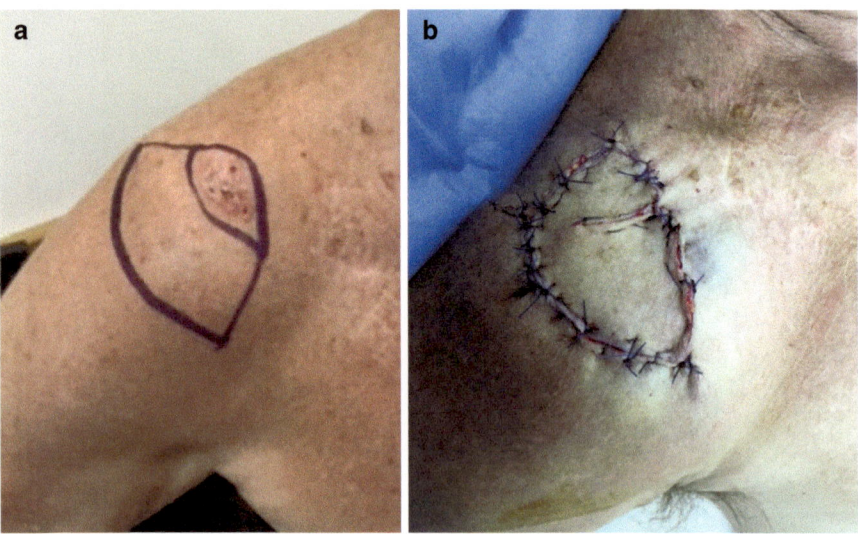

Fig. 13.13 Keystone flap (my latest example) used to repair a defect of the right shoulder following wide excision of a multifocal BCC (**a**). Adjacent scarring from previous surgery in this 64-year-old man necessitated the Omega variant option. Immediate post-operative result (**b**)

Notes
Keystone flaps in the shoulder girdle region allow early mobilization and do not seem to produce hypertrophic or keloid scars.

Trunk

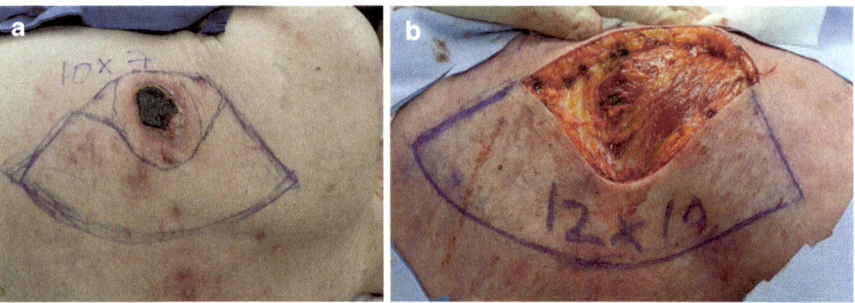

Fig. 13.14 Large keystone flap (Omega variant) for repair of left scapular defect in an 88-year-old man, following excision of a necrotic herpes zoster ulcer (**a–c**). Immediate post-operative result (**d**)

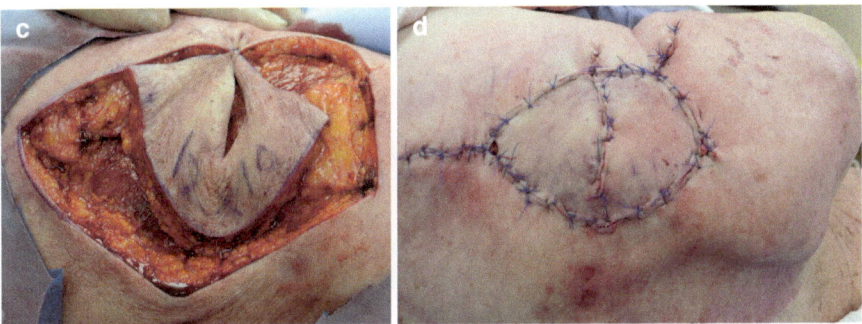

Fig. 13.14 (continued)

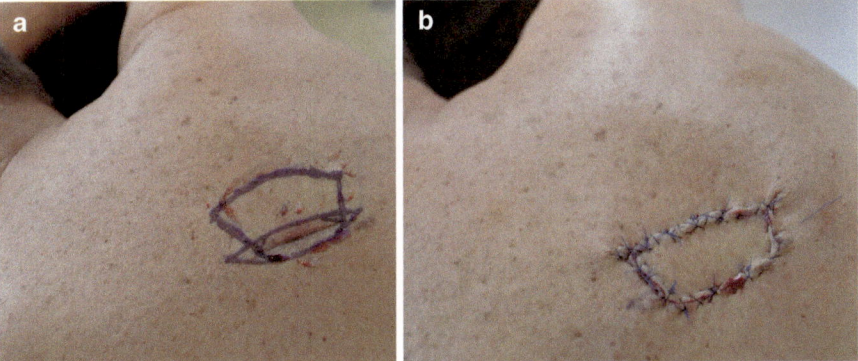

Fig. 13.15 A smaller keystone flap (classical version) was used for the right scapular region of a 54-year-old man following wider excision of a melanoma in situ (**a, b**)

Notes
Like the keystone flaps for the shoulder region, trunk keystone flaps allow for early mobilization, and are surprisingly relatively painless in the post-operative phase.

Lower Limb

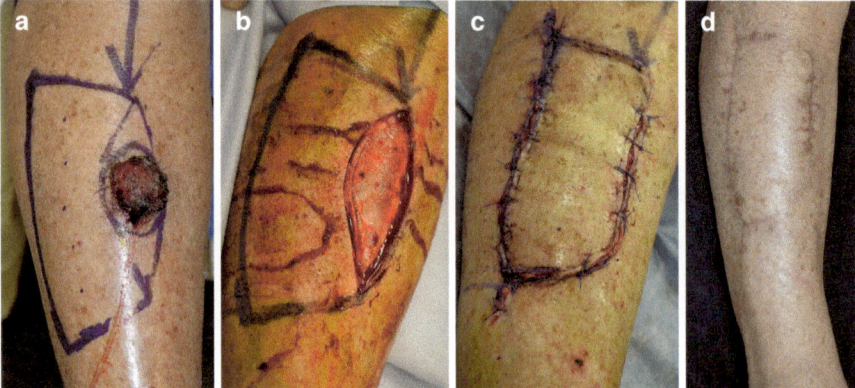

Fig. 13.16 Wide excision of a keratoacanthoma arising on the right shin of a 67-year-old woman and repair with a large keystone flap based on the perforators of the peroneal muscle compartment (**a–c**). The result at 4 months (**d**)

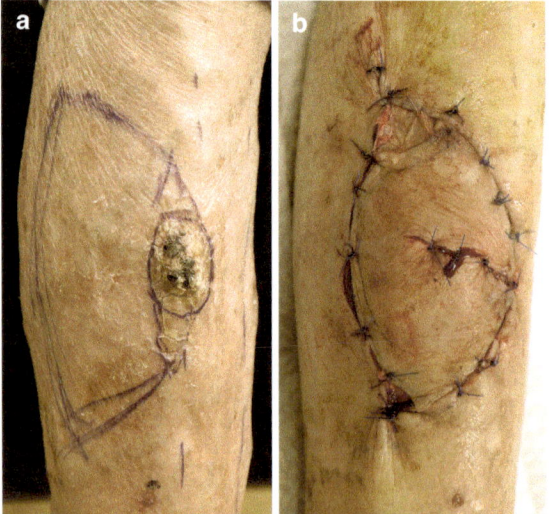

Fig. 13.17 A well-differentiated SCC on the anterior shin of a 96-year-old man widely excised and repaired with a keystone flap (Omega variant) with small split skin graft to the proximal secondary defect (**a, b**). Result at 2 years (**c**). (**d**) This illustrates the concept of the Omega variant for the keystone perforator island flap. The lateral thirds of the flap are undermined in the subcutaneous plane, with mobilization in an Omega configuration so that points *A* and *B* converge on *C*. The resulting dog-ear (*triangular image*) is excised still preserving the island pedicle supplying the flap complex. The superior and inferior segments will need skin grafting or heal by secondary intention

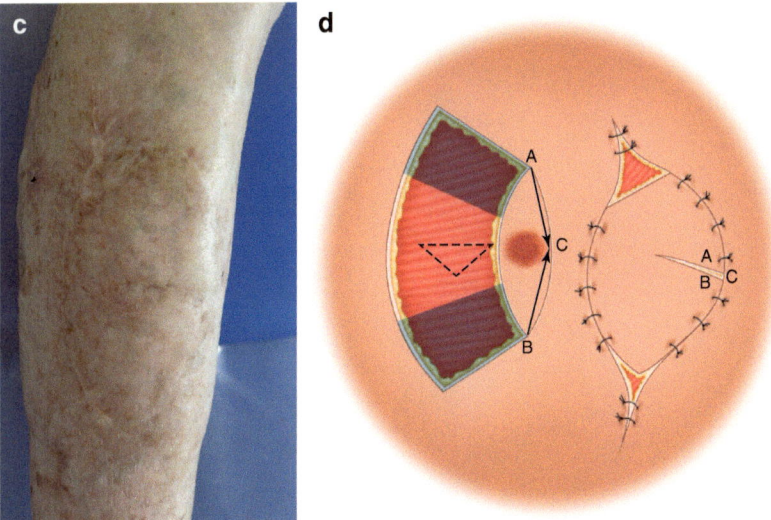

Fig. 13.17 (continued)

Notes

Keystone flaps have made significant changes to how I repair defects on the lower limb, especially in my older patients. Skin grafts are now the exception, and the keystone local flap has become a preferred option. Be particularly careful of the patients with thin atrophic skin, diabetes mellitus and those on anticoagulation. The flaps must be dissected precisely and the wounds closed very loosely. An example of this is given in Chap. 3 on technical tips.

Hand

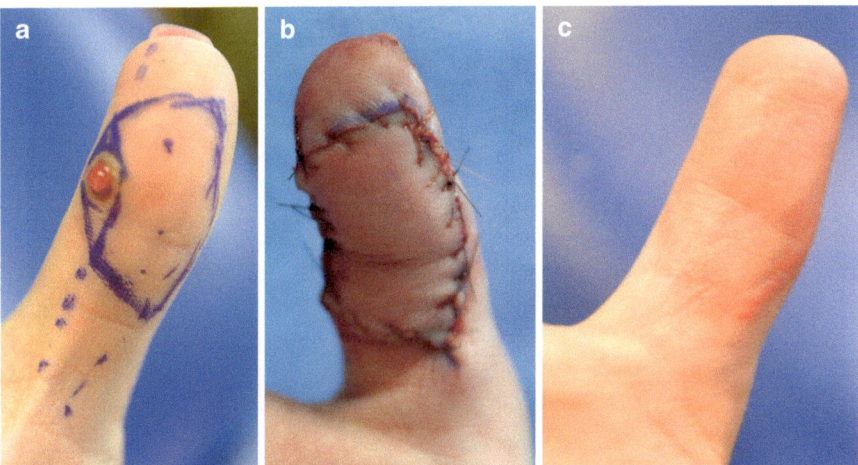

Fig. 13.18 A keystone flap was used to close the radial defect of the thumb of a 26-year-old woman with diabetes, following excision of a painful pyogenic granuloma (**a**, **b**). Full sensation was retained in the finger. Result at 4 months (**c**)

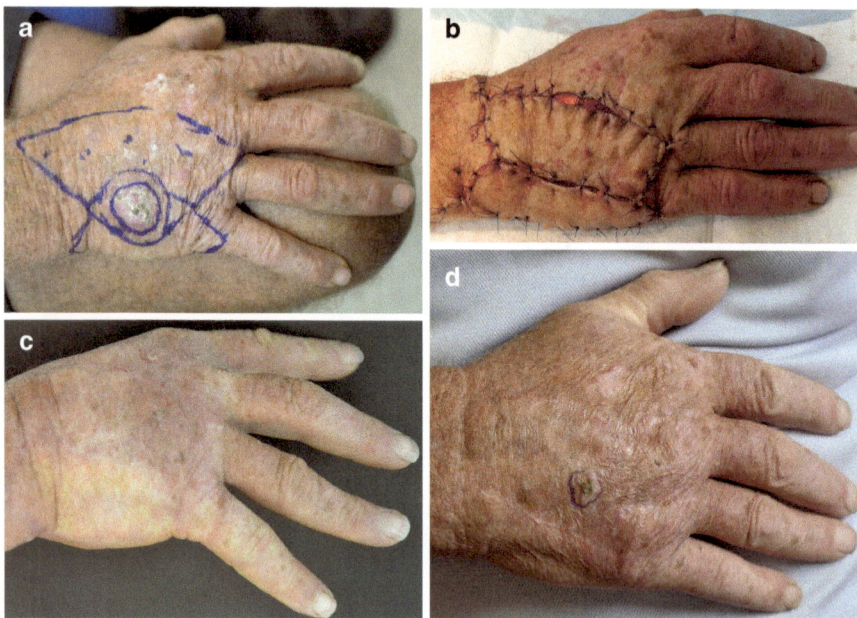

Fig. 13.19 Wide excision of an SCC arising on the dorsum of a 68-year-old man's right hand (**a**) and repair with double keystone local flaps (**b**). Result at 4 months (**c**) and 2 years (**d**) when he presented again with a superficial lichenoid solar keratosis on one of the flaps

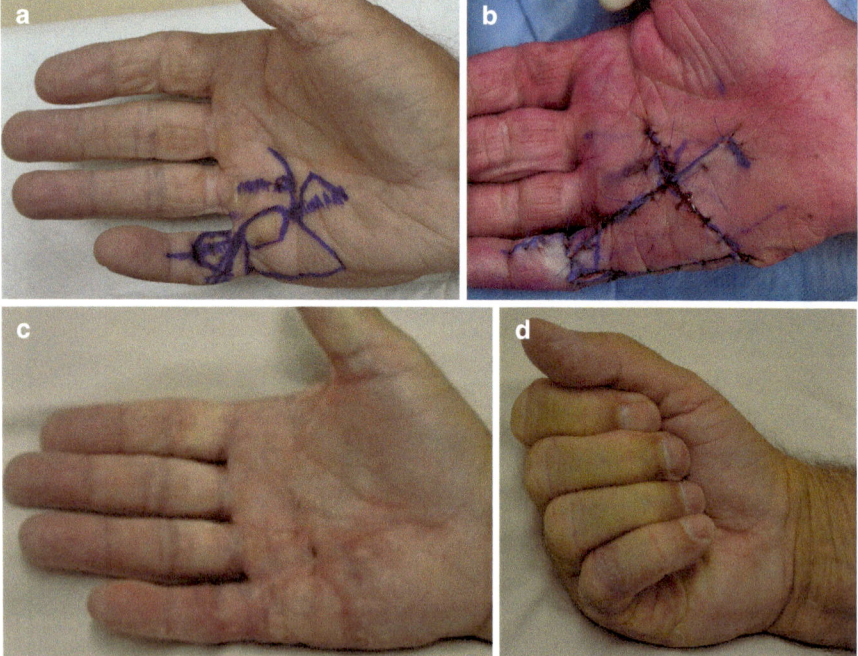

Fig. 13.20 Keystone flap at the base of the right little finger designed to repair the palmar skin defect following dermofasciectomy for Dupuytren's palmar fibromatosis in a 61-year-old man (**a**, **b**). Result at 6 weeks (**c**, **d**)

Notes

Keystone flaps in the hand heal rapidly, and hand function is preserved because the patient can gently mobilise whilst healing proceeds. This is particularly important after the extensive hand and digit dissection associated with Dupuytren's surgery.

Foot

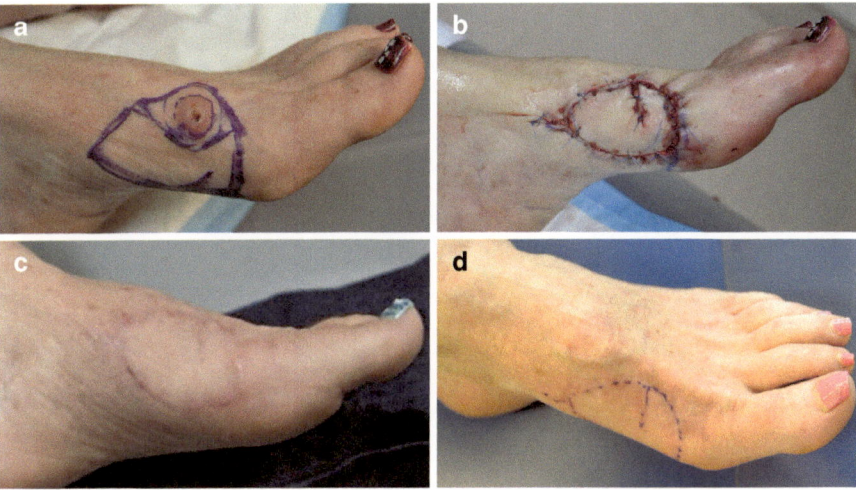

Fig. 13.21 Keystone local flap (Omega variant) for the defect on the medial aspect of a 55-year-old woman's left forefoot, following wide excision of a SCC (**a, b**). Result at 4 months (**c**) and 2 years (**d**) with flap edges highlighted using a marking pen

Combination Flaps

Keystone Advancement + Chin Rotation Flaps

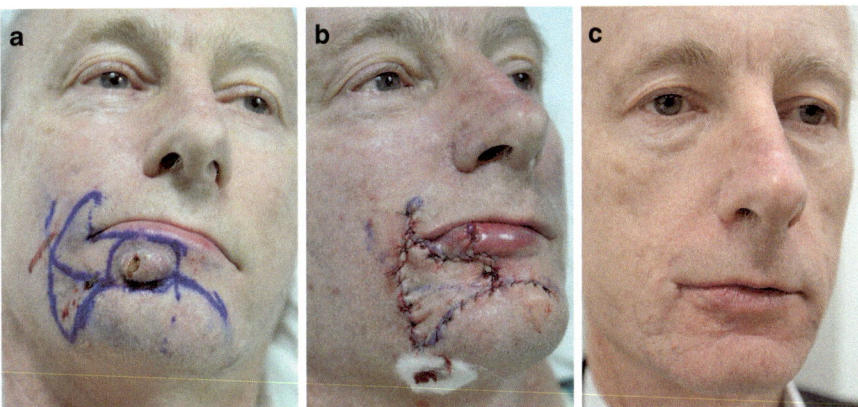

Fig. 14.1 Keratoacanthoma on the lower lip/chin junction of a 55-year-old man. Excision completed with 5 mm margins and the defect repaired with a perioral keystone perforator island local flap from the right side and an inferiorly based chin rotation flap from the left (**a**, **b**). Wedge resection of right lower lip dog-ear required. Result at 9 months (**c**)

© Springer International Publishing AG 2018
M.F. Klaassen et al., *Simply Local Flaps*,
https://doi.org/10.1007/978-3-319-59400-2_14

Notes

Oral competence is the key function to preserve in this reconstruction of the lower lip and respect for the resting skin tension lines. Balance of the vermillion lip contours is also important, and sometimes a mucosal revision is required to remove excess mucosal tissue.

Cervicofacial Rotation + Glabellar Transposition Flaps

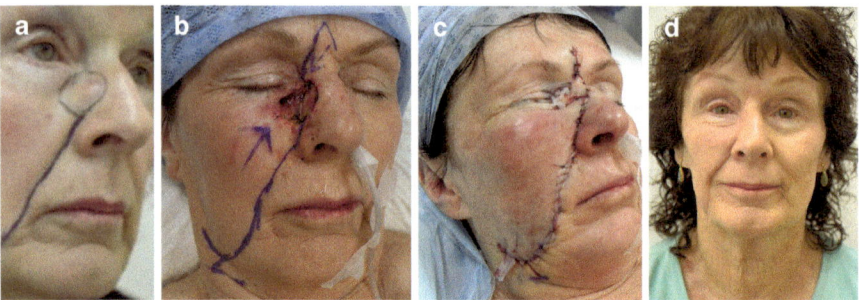

Fig. 14.2 A right nasojugal tumour of uncertain origin (ruptured dermoid cyst), in this 67-year-old woman (**a**) widely excised and reconstruction delayed for 24 h, awaiting urgent histology (**b**). The defect involving the right nasojugal and lateral nasal subunits, was repaired with a cervicofacial rotation flap, combined with a glabellar transposition flap (**c**). The result at 3 months (**d**)

Notes

Extra length can be added to the cheek rotation flap with the addition of a Z-plasty at the jawline as illustrated in Figs. 14.2b and 14.2c.

Forehead Interpolated Flap + Cheek Rotation Flap + Lip Switch Flap

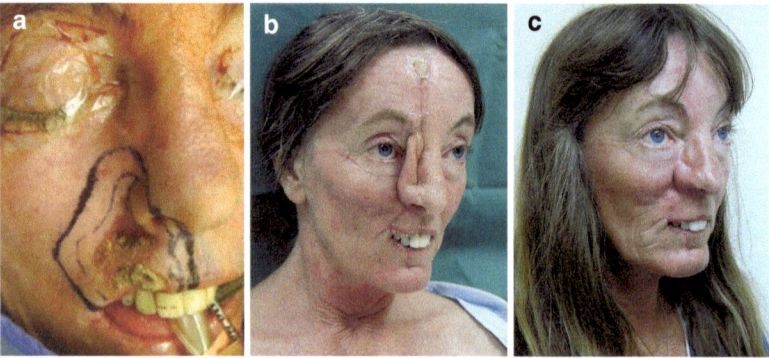

Fig. 14.3 (**a–c**): An extensive ulcerated BCC in a young woman treated elsewhere with antibiotics for some months. The infiltrating BCC involved the right upper lip, alar base and medial cheek (**a**). Staged reconstruction was performed after wide and complete margin-controlled excision with a right lower lip-switch flap and inferiorly based cheek rotation flap to provide a platform for the paramedian forehead flap alar reconstruction (**b**). The result after three stages at 1 year (**c**)

Combination Keystone Flaps from Cervical and Cheek Regions

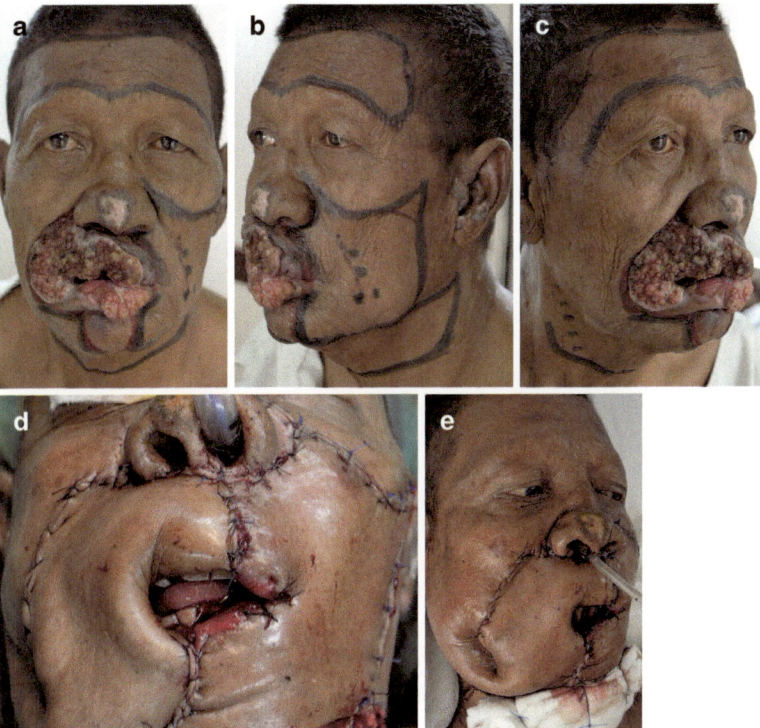

Fig. 14.4 This 45-year-old clergyman presented to our Interplast team in Port Moresby, Papua-New Guinea with an extensive fungating SCC of his mouth, secondary to chronic betel nut chewing (**a–c**). Transfer to New Zealand or Australia for care was not an option. A wide excision was undertaken with the local surgical team, and two keystone flaps (right cervicomental and left cheek) for cover plus a potential total forehead flap for lining were planned (**a–c**). The forehead flap was ultimately not required as the large cervicomental keystone flap based on right sternomastoid perforators was folded to provide upper lip lining. The secondary neck defect was repaired with split skin graft but in hindsight could have been reconstructed with the supraclavicular flap of Lamberty. Immediate result shown (**d, e**). Long-term results are unavailable

Part IV

Judgement, Decision-making and Experience

Chapter 15: Where Skin Grafts Are Better

In reality sometimes a skin graft is a preferred reconstructive option and we add this to contrast the use of local flaps with that of skin grafts.

Chapter 16: Asthetica

This is not new but we define it as a useful concept; using methods developed in the practice of cosmetic surgery of the face for skin cancer defects.

Chapter 17: Complications: Their Management and Prevention

These are inevitable and must be managed with skill, judgement and sound decision-making. The lead author shares his management of some challenging complications, resulting from his use of local flaps in reconstruction.

Chapter 18: How to Think Like a Plastic Surgeon

We try to bring all the concepts and principles together by considering two selected clinical cases. These difficult cases are selected to define the standards of thinking required for success in the FRACS (Plast.) final fellowship exam.

Where Skin Grafts Are Better

15

Scalp

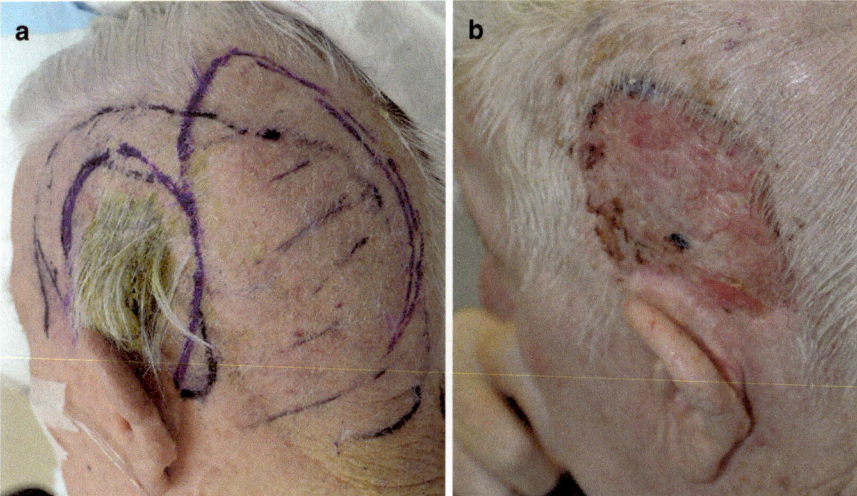

Fig. 15.1 A fungating SCC on the left parietal scalp of a 92-year-old man, arising from previous incompletely excised SCC in situ (**a**). The initial plan for an inferiorly based scalp transposition flap was abandoned, following wide excision of the SCC, in favour of a split skin graft. Result at 2 weeks (**b**)

© Springer International Publishing AG 2018
M.F. Klaassen et al., *Simply Local Flaps*,
https://doi.org/10.1007/978-3-319-59400-2_15

Frontal Region

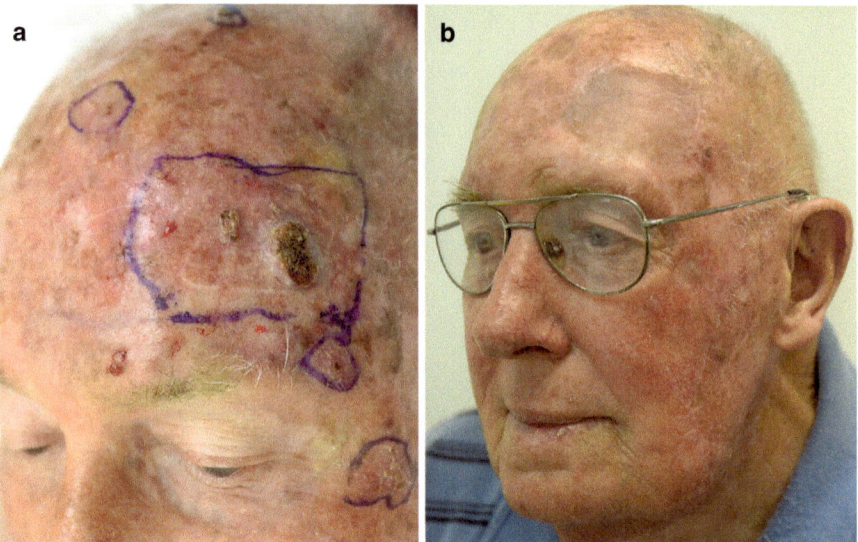

Fig. 15.2 A recurrent multifocal SCC on the solar damaged left forehead of this 86-year-old man (**a**) was widely excised and repaired with a supraclavicular full thickness skin graft. Satisfactory results at 5 months (**b**)

Nose

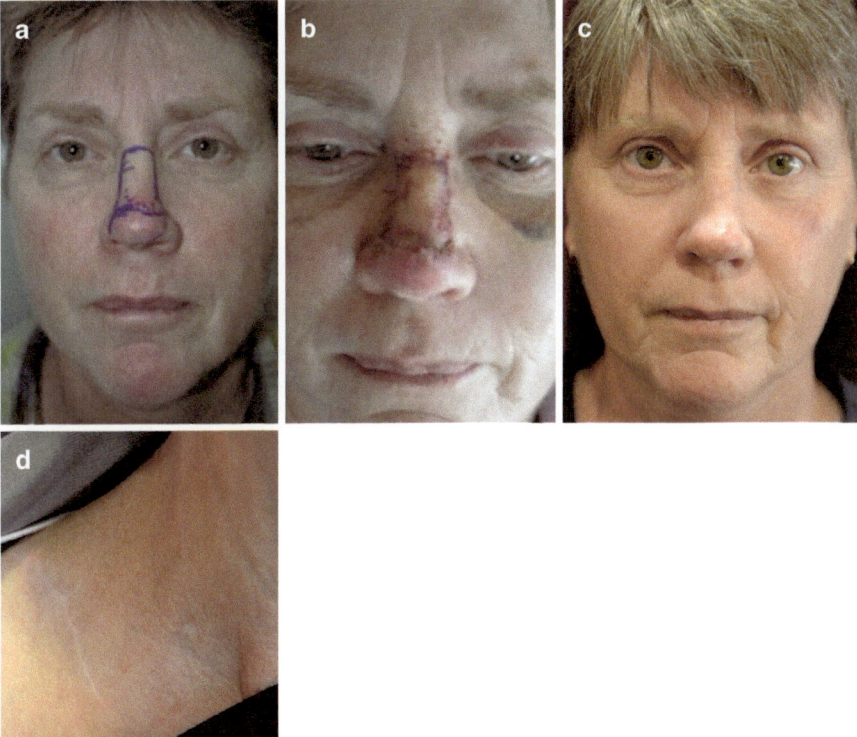

Fig. 15.3 A multifocal BCC on the dorsum of the nose in this 52-year-old woman was excised as a dorsal aesthetic subunit (**a**) and repaired with a supraclavicular full thickness skin graft. Results at 10 days (**b**) and 2 years (**c**). Appearance of the right supraclavicular donor scar at 1 year (**d**)

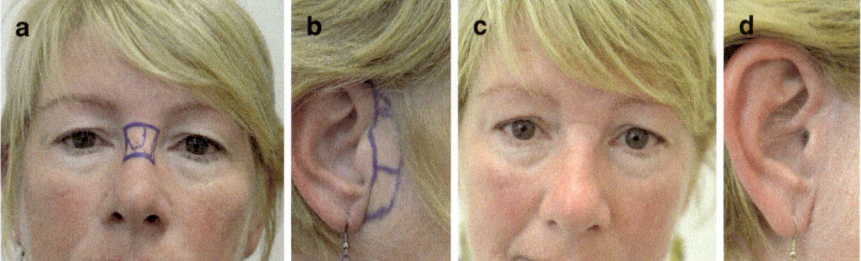

Fig. 15.4 A nodulocystic BCC of the nasal bridge of this 56-year-old woman was excised (**a**) and repaired with a preauricular full thickness skin graft (**b**). Results of the nose (**c**) and donor site (**d**), at 4 months

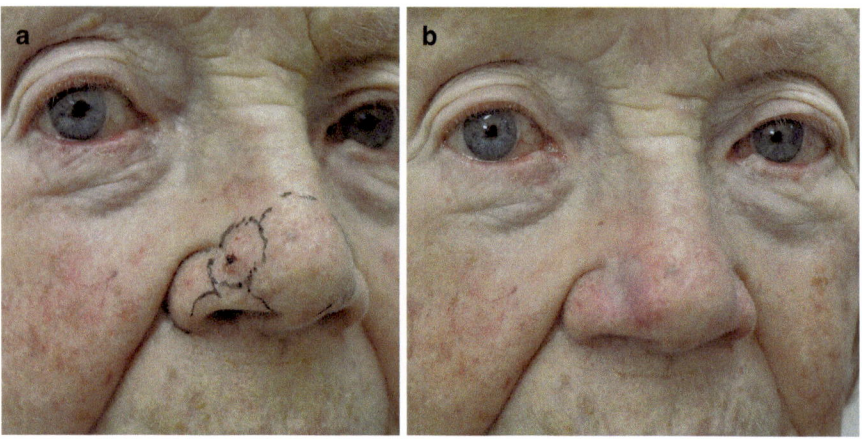

Fig. 15.5 A nodulocystic BCC on the right ala-nasal tip junction of the nose of an 83-year-old woman, was excised and repaired with a preauricular full thickness skin graft (**a**). Appearance at 4 months (**b**)

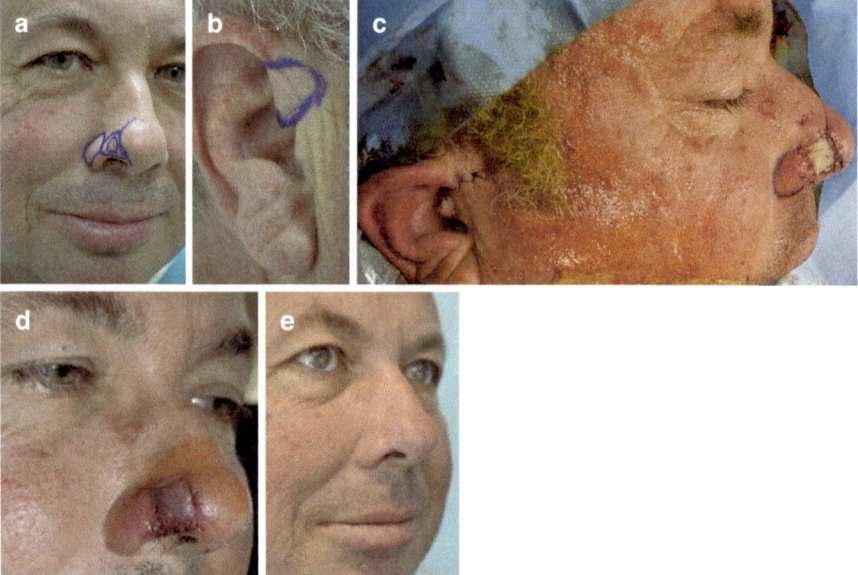

Fig. 15.6 An infiltrating BCC close to the right nostril rim in a 51-year-old man with type 2 diabetes mellitus was excised as a soft triangle aesthetic subunit (**a**). A composite graft taken from the right helical root (**b**) was used to reconstruct the full thickness defect (**c**). A de-epithelialised cephalad extension of the graft improved the graft take. The graft is revascularised at a week (**d**). Result at 2 years (**e**)

The Upper Lip

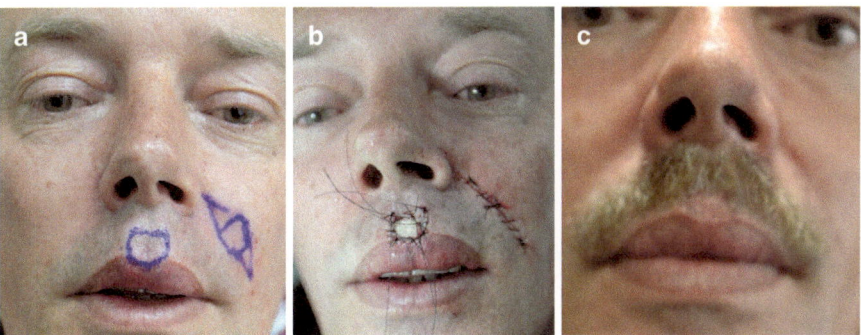

Fig. 15.7 A biopsy-proven infiltrating BCC of the central upper lip in this 43-year-old man was widely excised, and the defect was repaired with a full thickness skin graft from the left nasolabial fold region (**a, b**). Result at 4 weeks (**c**)

Notes

Full thickness skin grafts achieve a very good reconstruction on the face of older patients (>70 years). They can also give an excellent aesthetic reconstruction in younger patients, providing the donor site is selected with care.

There is plenty of spare full thickness skin in the neck regions of our elderly patients for donor skin.

The split skin graft ('old faithful') should never be left out of the reconstructive toolbox.

Harvesting a split (partial thickness) skin graft with the traditional Humby, Cobbett or Watson skin grafting knives is still mandatory for any competent plastic surgeon.

For the face, matching of colour and texture for an aesthetic graft repair is the key issue. Patience is also a virtue. The preauricular, postauricular, supraclavicular and nasolabial donor sites are best for small- to moderate-sized defects. For larger defects where a full thickness skin graft is selected, the inner arm is a useful donor site and can be closed directly.

Check for
updates

Aesthetica

16

It is important to define Aesthetica, because it is a new concept:

When the surgeon uses techniques developed in the practice of aesthetic surgery for reconstructive problems, the distinction between reconstructive and aesthetic surgery truly merges. It can be applied to the face, to the nose, to the breast and the abdomen (e.g. abdominoplasty method for closing the donor defect after TRAM or DIEP breast reconstruction). The facelift flap can be used to advance skin to repair defects of the preauricular, postauricular, zygomatic and temporal facial regions. Bilateral full thickness skin grafts can be harvested from the prauricular donor site and the defects closed as for a mini-facelift. There is an example of the serendipitous flap for conchal reconstruction with the donor site closed as for a mini-facelift (see Fig. 7.7 on page 77).

Bilateral Preauricular Skin Grafts

Classification: Large defects of the face requiring full thickness skin grafts. The donor sites are repaired directly as for a mini-facelift.

Clinical case scenario: This 55-year-old woman presented with three recurrent BCCs on her nose including the dorsum and lateral nasal sidewalls. She was motivated to have natural facial rejuvenation. I felt it worth saving the forehead flap option for future reconstructive needs. The lesions were removed as nasal aesthetic subunits and repaired with preauricular skin grafts removed during a mini-facelift.

© Springer International Publishing AG 2018

M.F. Klaassen et al., *Simply Local Flaps*,

https://doi.org/10.1007/978-3-319-59400-2_16

Fig. 16.1 Mini-facelift simulation manoeuvre

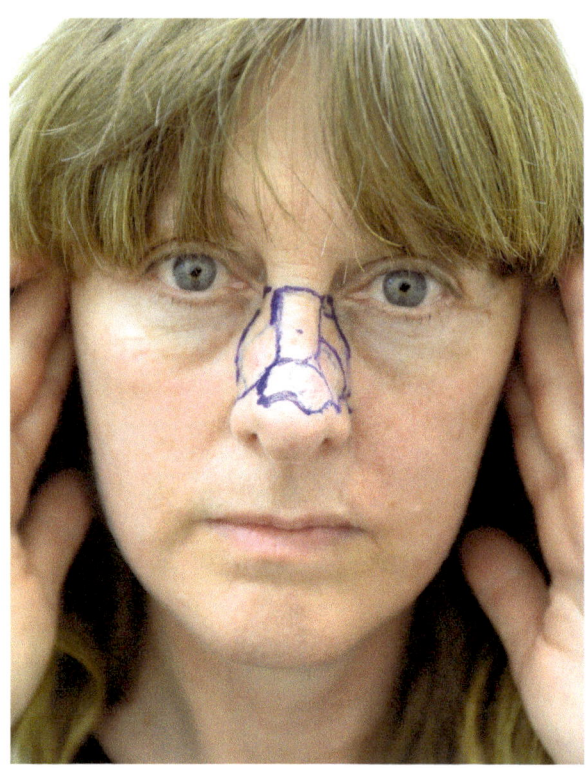

Notes

Patients need to be informed that their facial appearance will change with the mini-facelift, but this will look natural in the medium term. It is important to demonstrate this to them with the facelift simulation manoeuvre in front of a mirror (see Fig. 16.1).

After the preauricular skin graft harvest, judicious undermining of the lateral cheeks is performed with facelift scissors or sharp scalpel to aid a tensionless closure of the preauricular wounds. Dermal pennant flaps (as described by Dr. Lawrence Ho, FRACS) planned in the residual preauricular skin are de-epithelialised and anchored to the postauricular cartilage [2]. This improves the final scar and avoids distortion of the ear lobes. Donor sites are closed as for the skin only facelift. SMAS plication may be performed, but in Fig. 16.2, it was not.

The face will feel tight, and I advise patients to have a soft diet and take regular analgesia for the first week or two after surgery. Prof. Jim Frame of England recommends patients should wear a soft cervical splint as well, for splintage of the rejuvenated face over the first 2 weeks.

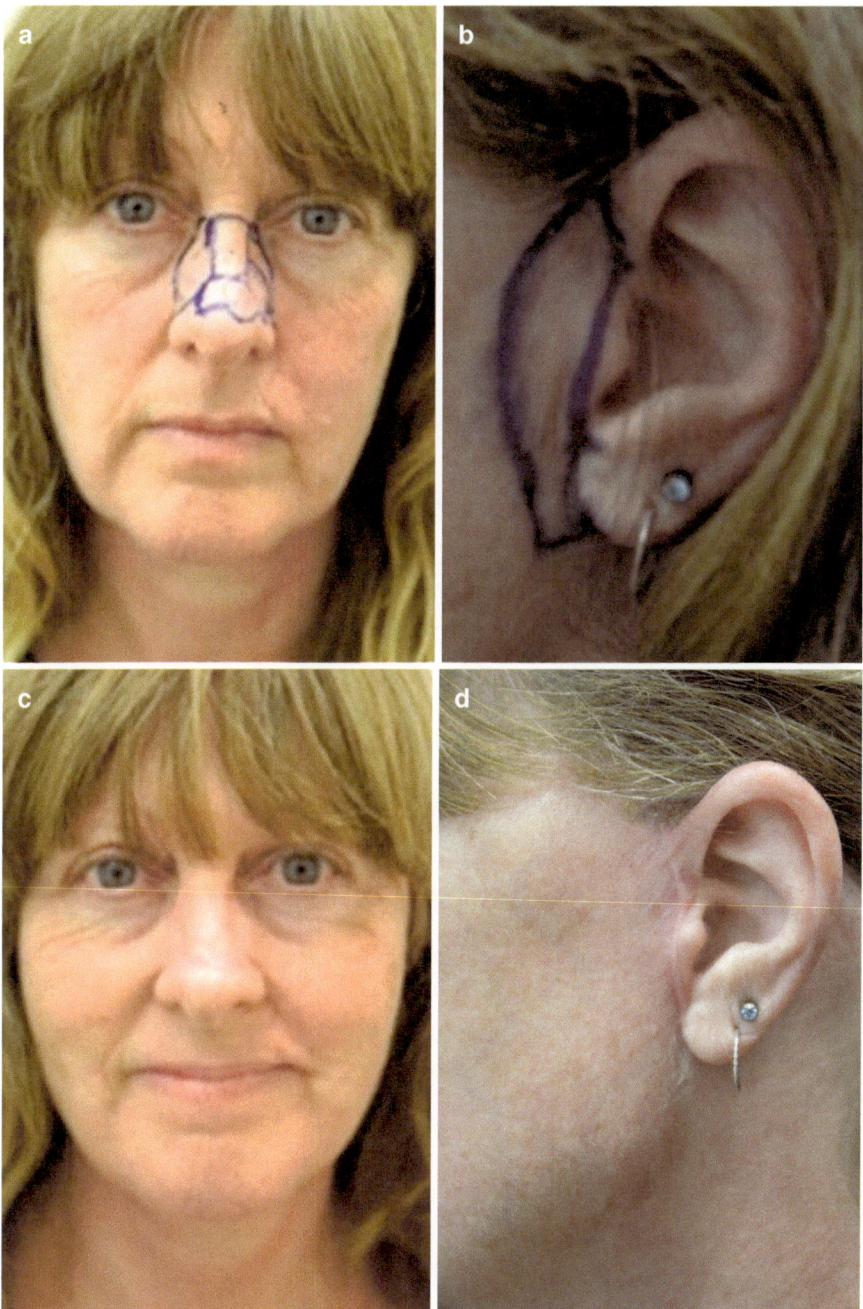

Fig. 16.2 Recurrent BCCs of the dorsum and sidewalls of the nose of a 55-year-old woman were removed as nasal aesthetic subunits (**a**) and repaired with two preauricular full thickness skin grafts (**b**). Results of the nose (**c**) and donor site (**d**) at 8 months

Facelift flaps

Type I: Mini Preauricular Facelift Flaps

Classification: Advancement/broad-based /single stage

Clinical case scenario: An ulcerated atypical fibroxanthoma on the root of the right helix in a 69-year-old man

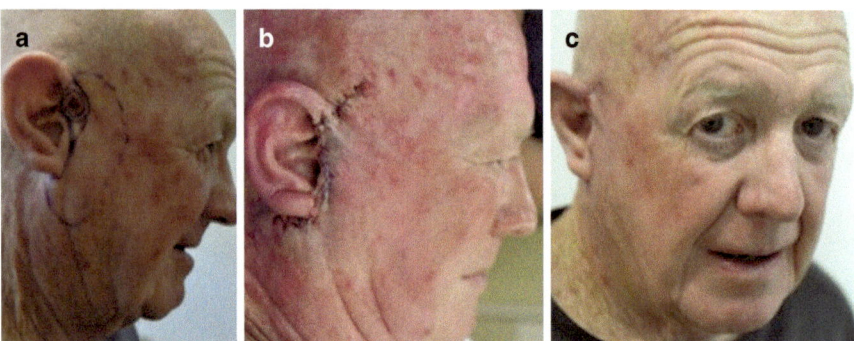

Fig. 16.3 An atypical fibroxanthoma in a 69-year-old man (**a**) excised and repaired with a mini preauricular facelift flap (**b**). Result at 2 weeks (**c**)

Notes
This is a straightforward reconstruction under local anaesthetic. The extent of the preauricular undermining is indicated in Fig. 16.3a. A tension-less closure is achieved with undermining and Dr. Ho's dermal pennant flaps.

Type 2: Moderate Preauricular Facelift Flap

Classification: Advancement/broad-based/single stage

Clinical case scenario: A large nodulocystic basal cell carcinoma on the left temple of a 55-year-old man with associated jawline actinic keratoses

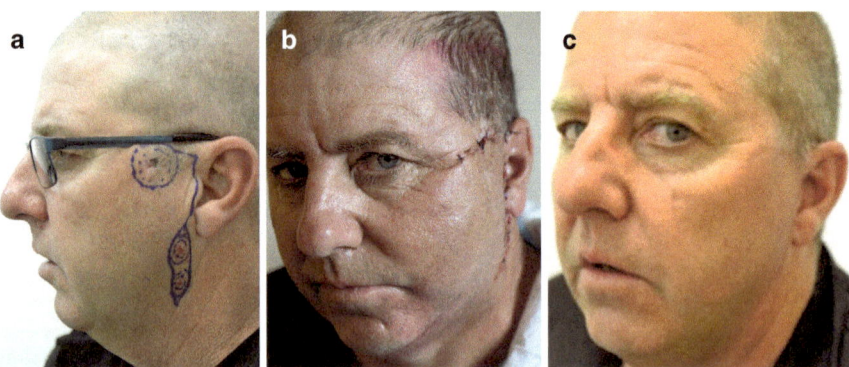

Fig. 16.4 A wide excision of left temple BCC, along with excision of keratoses on the jawline of a 55-year-old man (**a**) and repair with a moderate facelift flap (**b**). Vertical vectors for advancement. Result at 6 months (**c**)

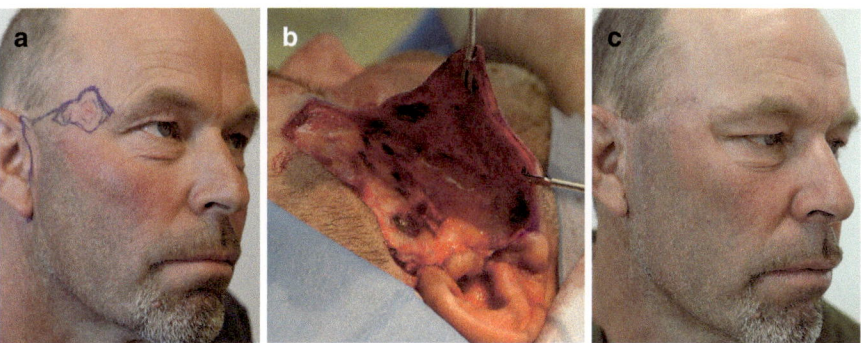

Fig. 16.5 A similar case to Fig. 16.4 of a BCC on the right zygomatic region of a 51-year-old man (**a**) was excised. The extent of facelift undermining (**b**) and result at 2 weeks (**c**)

Type 3: Extended Facelift Flap

Clinical case scenario: A large superficial basal cell carcinoma of the left postauricular/neck region with associated small BCC left zygomatic region

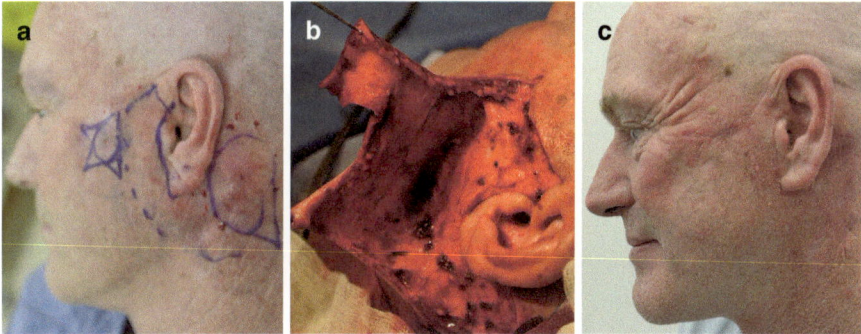

Fig. 16.6 A large multifocal superficial BCC left postauricular region in a 51-year-old man (**a**), excised and repaired with an extended (pre- and postauricular) facelift flap. Extent of undermining for the extended facelift flap (**b**) and result at 4 months (**c**)

Notes

At least 6 cm of undermining is required for the extended facelift flap. Drainage and pressure dressing is recommended for 24 hours following surgery.

Male patients tolerate this procedure very well under local anaesthetic, supplemented if necessary by intravenous sedation as a day case. The facelift flaps are very well vascularized. I always check the patients for haematoma within 24 hours.

Long-term facial asymmetry does not seem to be a problem.

References

1. Penington AJ (2012) Local flap reconstruction—a practical approach, 2nd edn. McGraw-Hill, Sydney
2. Ho LCY, Klaassen MF, Mithraratne K. (2018), The Congruent Facelift: a three-dimensional view. Springer Nature.

Complications: Their Management and Prevention

17

Haematoma

Classification: Early post-operative

Clinical case scenario: A 62-year-old man on low-dose aspirin, with a recurrent basal cell carcinoma on the right temple, developed a painful haematoma under a rotation scalp flap 3 hours following surgery. He felt a 'pop' under the flap, developed active bleeding and attended the Emergency Department. A compression bandage was applied, but the haematoma was neither recognized nor drained. He re-presented the following morning.

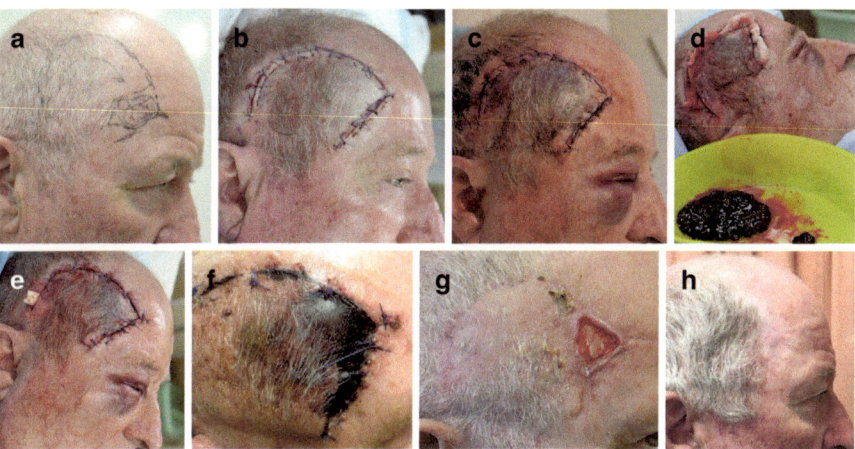

Fig. 17.1 A BCC on the right temple of a 62-year-old man (**a**) removed and repaired with a rotation scalp flap (**b**) presented with a haematoma under the scalp flap (**c**) which was not recognized. Evacuation of the haematoma was delayed (**d**), resulting in partial necrosis of the scalp flap (**e, f**). The necrotic flap was debrided and the wound healed by secondary intention over 6 weeks (**g**). Result at 2 years (**h**)

© Springer International Publishing AG 2018
M.F. Klaassen et al., *Simply Local Flaps*,
https://doi.org/10.1007/978-3-319-59400-2_17

Notes

Haematoma under a reconstructive flap is a surgical emergency. The pressure on the flap leads to ischaemic necrosis. Timely release and evacuation of the haematoma is the urgent surgical management. Often the site of bleeding is not found due to vascular spasm. The use of surgical drains should be seriously considered following extensive flap elevation, dead space or a high chance of post-operative bleeding.

Patients should leave the surgical facility with a provisional or definitive operative note, with post-operative instructions, warnings and contact details for the surgeon and staff. They should be encouraged to take these documents with them, if an emergency situation leads to them to an Emergency Department. I personally give patients post-operatively my mobile contact phone number.

We need to be aware that many of our patients in this modern era are taking long-term anticoagulation drugs including low dose Aspirin*, Warfarin*, Clopidogrel and Rivaroxaban. For skin surgery I am usually happy to leave the patient on the two former drugs*, but for those patients on more aggressive anticoagulants, consultation with the attending cardiologist or clinical haematologist is recommended.

Venous Ischaemia

Classification: Early post-operative

Clinical case scenario: A 78-year-old woman with ischaemic heart disease, a pacemaker and on warfarin anticoagulation presented with squamous cell carcinomas on her scalp. She remained on warfarin and underwent excisional surgery and repair with two keystone flaps. Some bleeding was noted post-operatively, and 5 days later, she was noted to have total necrosis of one flap, due to venous outflow ischaemia. The necrotic flap was excised and the wound repaired with a split skin graft.

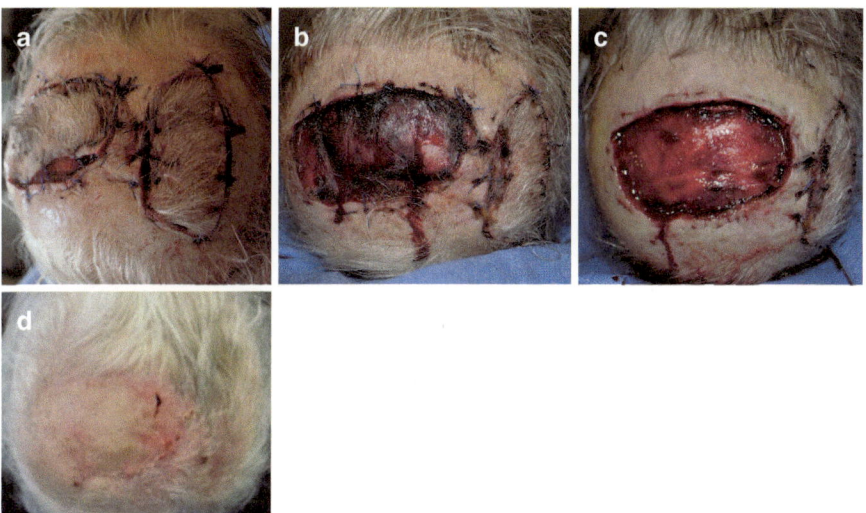

Fig. 17.2 Two keystone flaps on the scalp of a 78-year-old woman, following excision of SCCs (**a**). One flap developed necrosis with venous outflow ischaemia due to post-operative bleeding (**b**). At 7 days the obviously necrotic flap was debrided (**c**) and the wound repaired with a split skin graft. Result at 6 months (**d**)

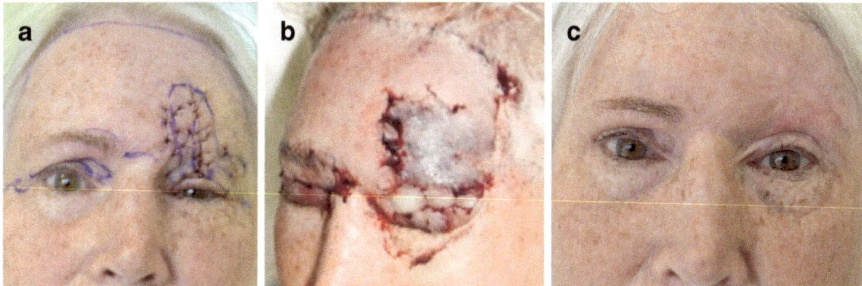

Fig. 17.3 A case similar to Fig.17.2. This patient had a wide excision, of a recurrent BCC and repair with a total forehead flap (**a**), which developed venous congestion (**b**) post-operatively. Result at 9 months following further surgery and a full thickness skin graft (**c**)

Radiation Necrosis

Classification: Late post-operative

Clinical case scenario: A 71-year-old man presented with a small squamous cell carcinoma on the antihelical fold of his left ear. Two years previously he received 60 Gy of radiation to the left parotid region for a metastatic squamous cell carcinoma of the left eyebrow. The superiorly based postauricular flap repair slowly necrosed over 3 weeks. Debridement, antibiotics and topical Flammazine were used to achieve healing.

Notes

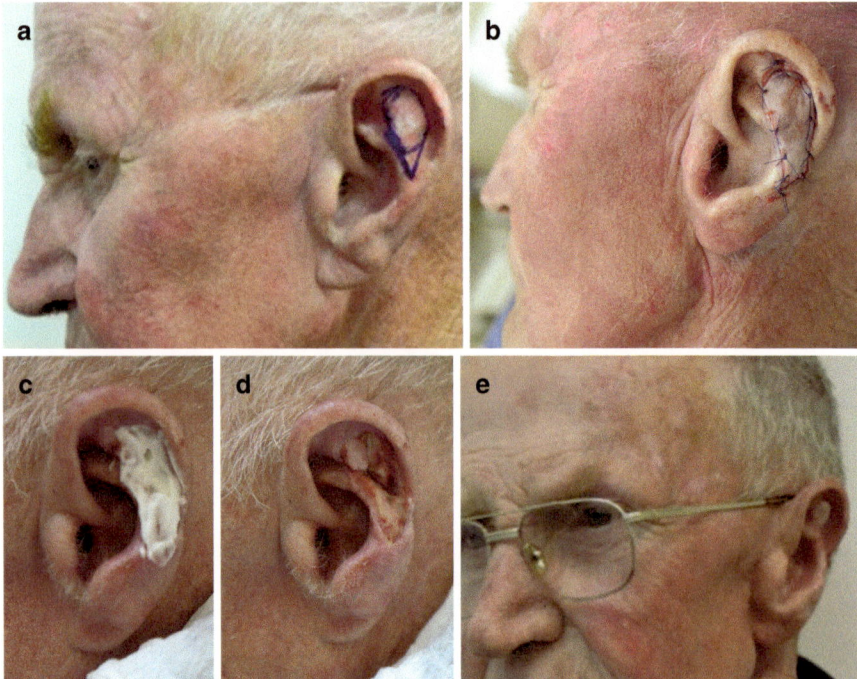

Fig. 17.4 An SCC on the antihelical fold of a 71-year-old man (**a**), excised and repaired with a superiorly based postauricular flap (**b**), which slowly necrosed, required debridement and topical Flammazine (**c**). Healing by secondary intention took 6 weeks (**d**). Result at 2 years (**e**)

A history of previous radiotherapy to a proposed donor site like the postauricular sulcus of the patient in Fig. 17.4 is a surgical red flag. Often there is no appearance of post-radiation skin damage. Consider other treatment options, because local flaps are at risk of late necrosis. Check the patient's file for the dose and type of radiation.

Secondary Viral Infection

Classification: Early post-operative

Clinical case scenario: A 38-year-old woman with a history of recurrent 'cold sores' required a vermilionectomy for actinic cheilitis of the lower lip. A severe herpes simplex infection was activated within 1 week of surgery. There was significant soft tissue inflammation and delayed healing, that resolved after antiviral medication.

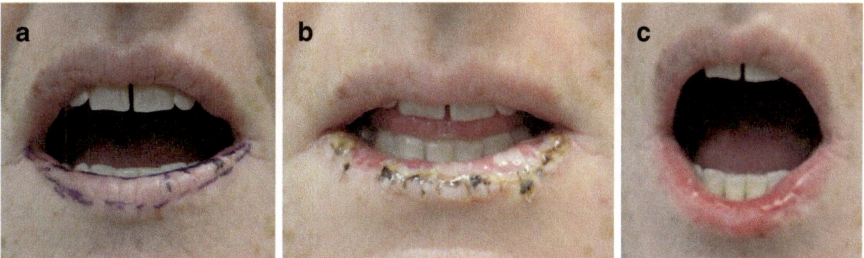

Fig. 17.5 Vermilionectomy was performed for severe dysplasia of the left lower lip in a 38-year-old woman (**a**). The patient developed a herpes simplex ulceration and inflammation within a week of surgery (**b**). This was treated with antiviral medication. Result at 8 weeks (**c**)

Hypertrophic Scars

Classification: Early—late post-operative

Clinical case scenario: A hypertrophic actinic keratosis was excised from the right cheek of this woman. The defect was repaired under no tension, with a sigmoid oblique advancement flap respecting the RSTLs. Persistent hypertrophic scarring resulted, which was treated with Micropore taping, massage and silicone gel.

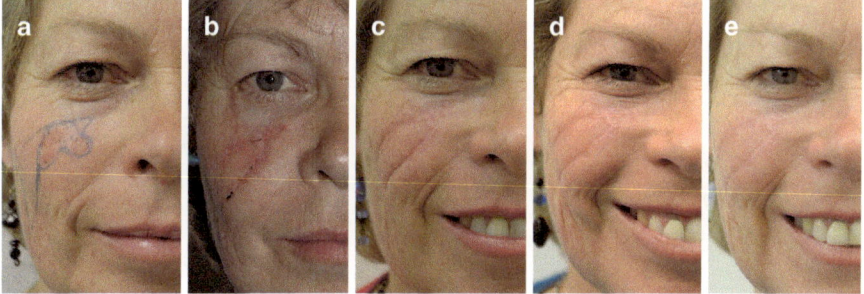

Fig. 17.6 A dysplastic hyperkeratotic actinic keratosis on the right cheek of a 50-year-old woman, excised and repaired with an Ono advancement flap (**a**, **b**), developed a persisting hypertrophic scar (**c**, **d**), which finally matured at 12 months (**e**)

Notes

It is important to discuss with patients before local flap surgery that scar quality varies from patient to patient, and the plastic surgeon does not have absolute control of the final scar.

A perfect scar is always the goal, but this may take time to mature and scar therapy is required with good patient compliance. The reasons for poor scars are considered and sound techniques applied to reduce the risk.

These include tensionless closure within relaxed skin tension lines, rapid healing without infection and gentle surgical technique. Leaving sutures in place for longer than necessary can leave marks that spoil the appearance of a beautiful flap repair.

Consider snipping the horizontal mattress sutures of a keystone flap after 2 weeks to prevent permanent suture marks.

The shoulder and presternal areas are 'danger zones for scars'. Surgery in these areas often produces hypertrophic or keloid scars, which may be very difficult to improve. Prevention and treatment strategies need to be considered. These include scar taping and silicone gel for prevention and then intra-lesional steroids or intra-lesional cryotherapy, for established hypertrophic or keloid scars.

Time is an important dimension in scar healing. Scar maturity may require some patience from both surgeon and patient.

For all new surgical scars, avoid prolonged UV light, which may cause hyperpigmentation during the first 6 months.

Ectropion Deformity

Classification: Early to medium post-operative

Clinical case scenario: An 85-year-old man with a recurrent multifocal basal cell carcinoma on his right medial cheek had an incipient cicatricial ectropion. This was aggravated by the reconstruction with a cheek rotation flap. He was treated with a full release of the ectropion and a full thickness skin graft.

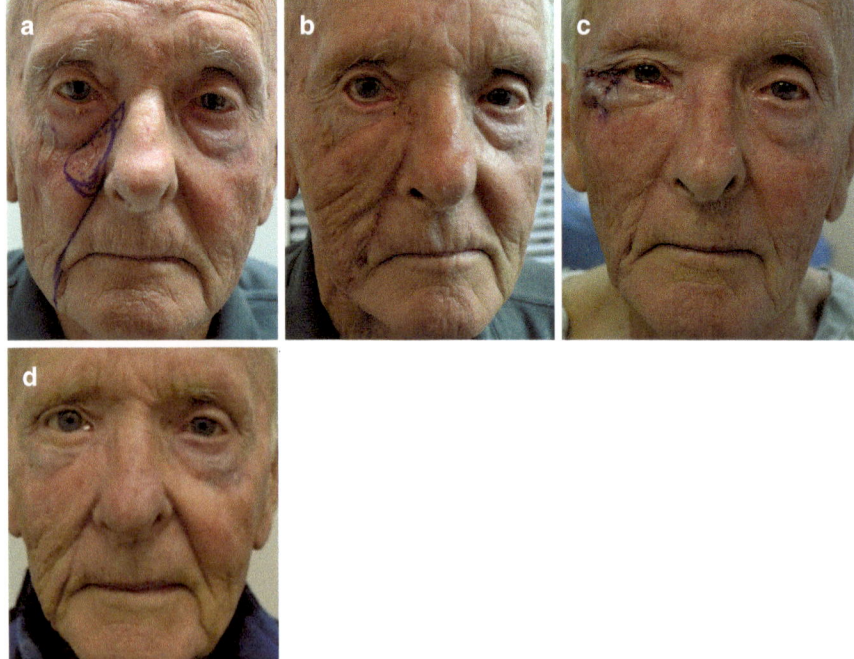

Fig. 17.7 A recurrent BCC on the medial upper right cheek of an 85-year-old man with incipient presurgery ectropion (**a**) was excised and the defect repaired with a rotation cheek flap. This caused an established right lower eyelid malposition (**b**). Result at 4 months following lateral tarsectomy (**c**) and 9 months following release of ectropion and full thickness skin graft (**d**)

Notes

Beware of the elderly patient with lower eyelid laxity and the risk of ectropion. A good examination technique is the lower eyelid snap test, as well as getting your patient to look upwards and watch what happens to the lower eyelids.

Another salvage repair option for the ectropion in Fig. 17.7 would have been a dermal sling procedure.

Oncological Issues

Oncological considerations are fairly obvious. Complete excision of a skin cancer is mandatory. More aggressive tumours require greater excision margins. If there is any doubt, then delayed reconstruction should be the plan. Frozen section tissue examination, controlled margin excision and urgent histology within 24 hours of surgery are all strategies available when collaborating with the local pathologists.

A temporary dressing or split skin graft will protect the wound bed, until the pathology report is confirmed. Margin-controlled tumour excision is a method we use in one of my clinics, because we have the proximity and collaborative relationship with the pathology laboratory. It is helpful for the histopathologist to have the specimen orientated with a suture. I tend to suture the 12 o'clock point as you view the specimen anatomically.

Risk Awareness and Consent

Know the potential complications of local flap surgery, and try to minimize them by correct diagnosis, a careful surgical plan and gentle surgical technique. Some complications may be managed conservatively, but others need reoperation. The timing of this is critical, and we are reminded of the principle of Gillies: *Don't do today what can honorably be put off until tomorrow.*

I tell all my patients, that if they are unlucky, a complication may occur. It is not the complication per se, as much as how the complication is recognized, accepted and managed, which is critical to the process of surgery. The patient with a complication should become your best friend. Be available and take full responsibility. You may even be forgiven!

How to Think Like a Plastic Surgeon

18

Case A

Classification: A complex defect involving the lateral right upper and lower eyelids

Clinical case scenario: A 91-year-old man, 4 months following a mild stroke, taking clopidogrel anticoagulant and referred with an infiltrating basal cell carcinoma of his right lateral canthus

On history this was a well-established lesion of at least 12 months duration, biopsy-proven nodular BCC with no morphoeic features. His right eye was his best eye for vision.

The examination confirmed a 3 × 2 cm infiltrating BCC, which was not fixed to the lateral orbital margin, but very close to the lateral canthus and eyelids. He also had an ulcerated BCC on the concha fossa of his right ear.

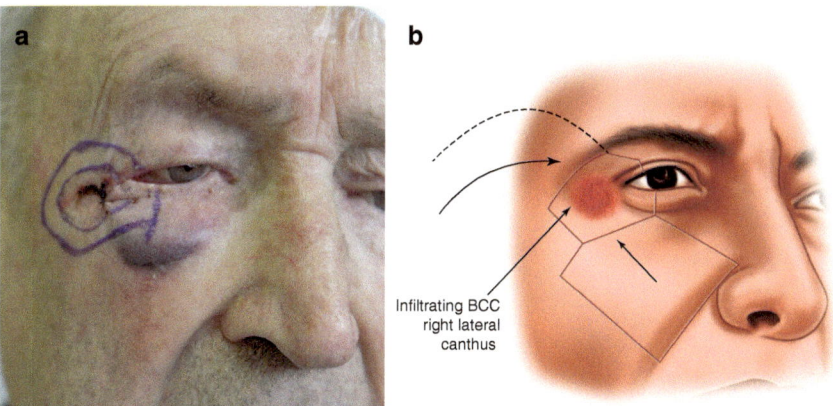

Infiltrating BCC right lateral canthus

Fig. 18.1 The problem: a 3 × 2 cm infiltrating BCC, lateral canthal region in a 91-year-old man, taking anticoagulants (**a**). The initial drawings for surgical plan illustrate initial reconstructive thoughts and options (**b**)

© Springer International Publishing AG 2018
M.F. Klaassen et al., *Simply Local Flaps*,
https://doi.org/10.1007/978-3-319-59400-2_18

Surgical management under local anaesthetic with sedation seemed appropriate, and he was asked to stop the clopidogrel 7 days before the procedure.

The important goals were patient safety, adequate excision margins, eyelid preservation and corneal protection, plus one-stage immediate reconstruction with local flaps and cartilage grafts for support.

The key questions to be considered in Case A are:

1. How much upper and lower eyelid will need to be resected?
2. How to reconstruct the lateral canthus?
3. What tissues are required to be replaced: conjunctiva, tarsal support and skin?
4. What are the sources of reconstructive tissue?

   Lining from conjunctival flaps or a chondro-mucosal graft from nasal septum
   Support from cartilage grafts from ear
   Cover from cheek flaps (rotation + keystone), supraorbital and temporal flaps

5. Adequate histology clearance of the BCC.
6. Single or staged surgical procedures?
7. Simultaneous excision and reconstruction of right concha?
8. What are the complication risks with the patient taking anticoagulants?
9. What is the lifeboat plan?
10. Private or public surgical facility?

Later, when recovering at home, he started bleeding. He was admitted to a local Emergency Department observation ward and discharged the following day.

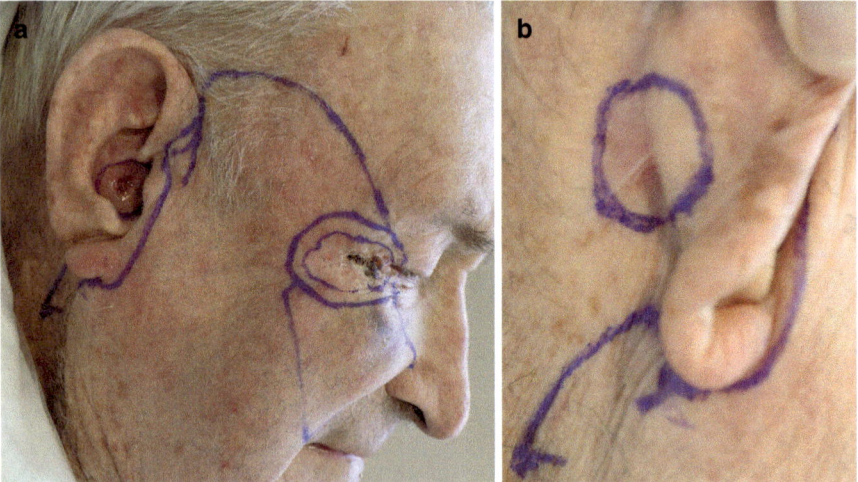

Fig. 18.2 Final excision plan with local flaps marked for periorbital (**a**) and conchal reconstruction (**b**)

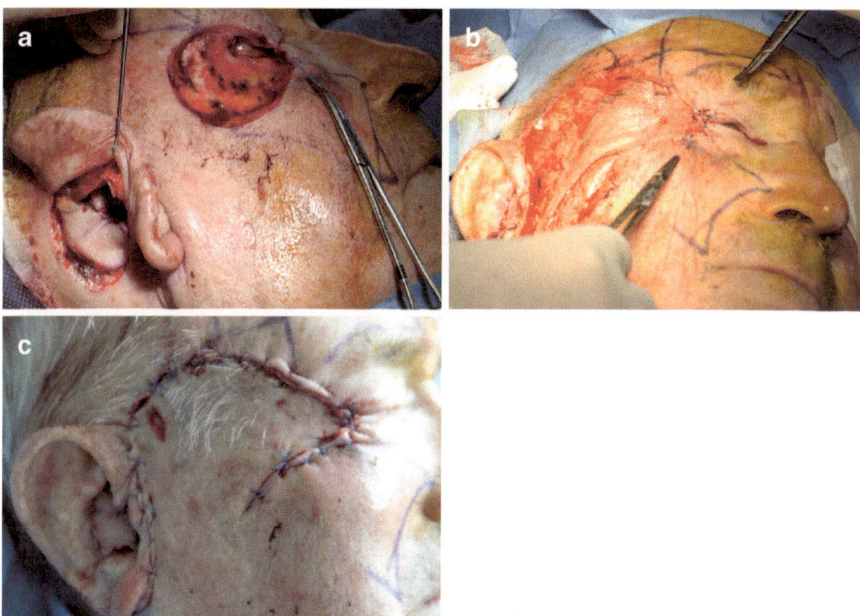

Fig. 18.3 Immediate reconstruction of the right periorbital and right conchal ear defects after complete excision of both tumours (**a, b**). Immediate post-operative result (**c**)

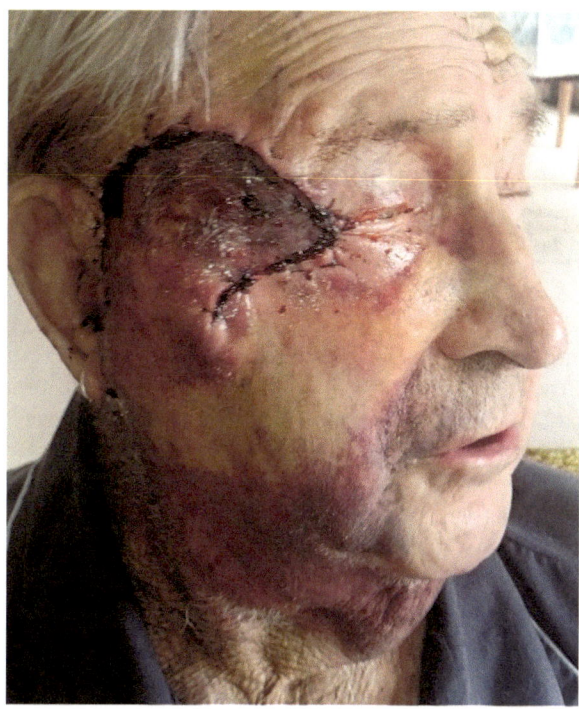

Fig. 18.4 The appearance of the patient the next day after several hours of observation in the local Emergency Department. The patient failed to take his provisional operative note and my contact details. No on-call surgeons were consulted by the emergency medical team.

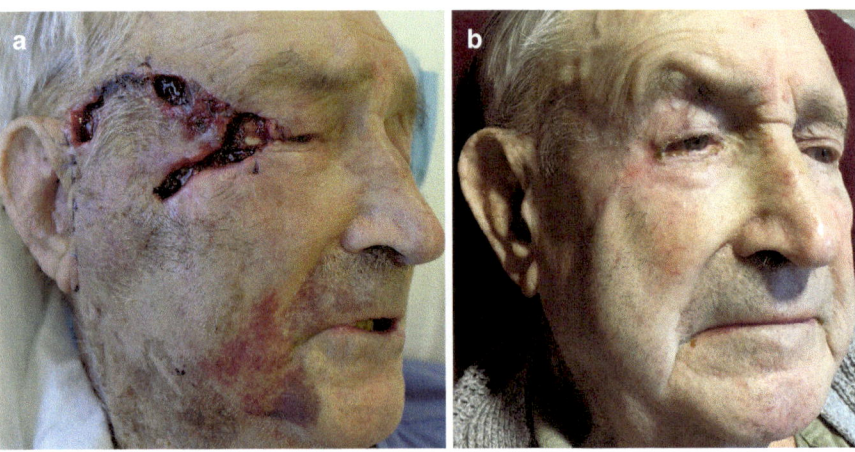

Fig. 18.5 (**a, b**) The haematoma under the rotation flap was evacuated, and some debridement of the flap edges was performed (**a**). Result at 3 months, with no sign of recurrence (**b**)

When examined by me the day after surgery, he was noted to have a haematoma and some marginal flap necrosis. The haematoma under the rotation flap was evacuated, and some debridement of the flap edges was required. He had several weeks of daily dressings, antibiotics and expert nursing care. The residual wounds healed by secondary intention with this regime after 2 months.

Notes

Bleeding and haematoma post-operatively are a real problem. Would a surgical drain have prevented the haematoma? Would hospital admission overnight help avoid this? I am not sure. It depends on the skill set of the other personnel outside your team, who become involved.

With healing by secondary intention, hypergranulation can become a problem, and here the silver nitrate stick is very useful.

Case B

Classification: A complex defect of the left nasal vestibule including columella and caudal septum

Clinical case scenario: A 75-year-old woman was referred with a T2 poorly differentiated squamous cell carcinoma of her left nasal vestibule.

On history, this was a painful ulcer of her left nasal vestibule treated with antibiotics for 3 months. She was a heavy smoker.

On examination, the ulcer measured 15 mm wide and arose from the left caudal septum with destruction of the columella but not extending into the right nasal vestibule.

Fig. 18.6 The problem, a penetrating poorly differentiated SCC of the caudal septum and columella

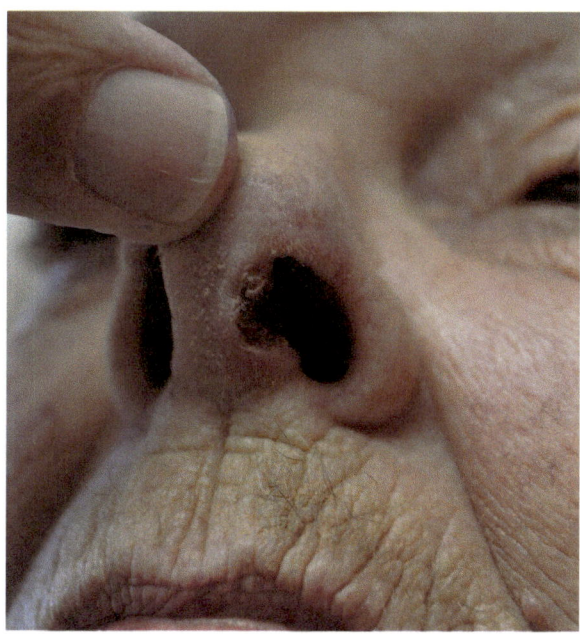

The surgical management was to perform a wide excision biopsy and to stage her disease. It proved to be a T2 lesion with no sign of regional or distant metastases. She stopped smoking immediately the diagnosis was made.

The **key questions** to be answered were:

1. What excision margin is oncologically acceptable?
2. Can we preserve her nasal form and function long term?
3. Will radiation therapy play a role?
4. How many stages of reconstruction will it take?
5. What problems can we expect from her smoking history?
6. How can we support her through this long process?
7. What are our lifeboats for complications?
8. Public or private surgical facility?
9. Multidisciplinary head and neck team involvement?

This patient's smoking history provided some challenges for healing, and several smaller surgical stages were required.

For the next 12 months, this patient had 8 stages of reconstruction with a 2-month gap between stages for her recovery. The tumour margins were all clear, and radiation therapy was considered but declined.

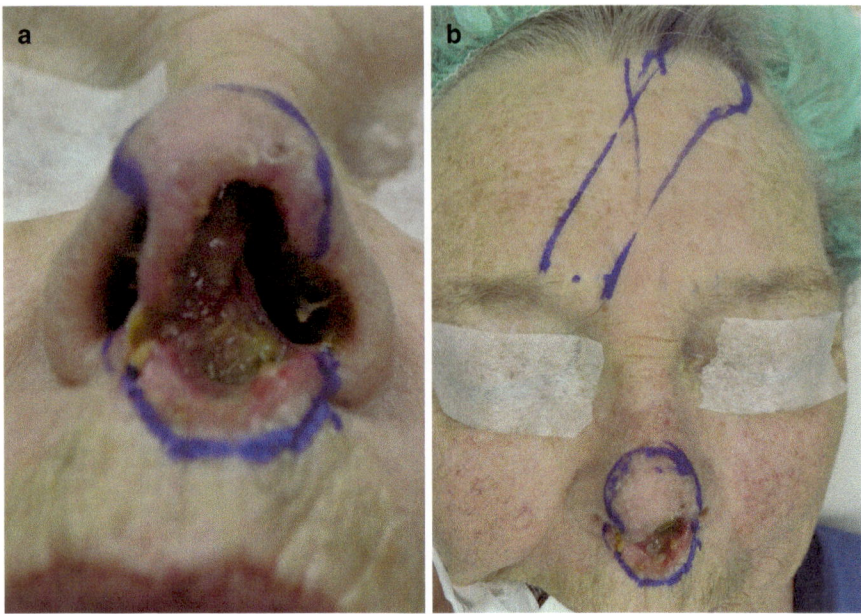

Fig. 18.7 Surgical plan for wide excision of nasal tip – columella – upper lip complex (**a**) and staged reconstruction (**b**)

Notes

This three-dimensional nasal reconstruction really does define plastic surgery and the use of local flaps.

'Like for like' as Sir Harold Gillies would say.

'Perfection is only just good enough', Sir William Manchester would add.

'Connection with your patient equals confident patient', Sir Archibald McIndoe would remind us.

We sit on the shoulders of the giants of our profession and carry on the legacy.

The good physician treats the disease; the great physician treats the patient who has the disease.

                                                                              William Osler

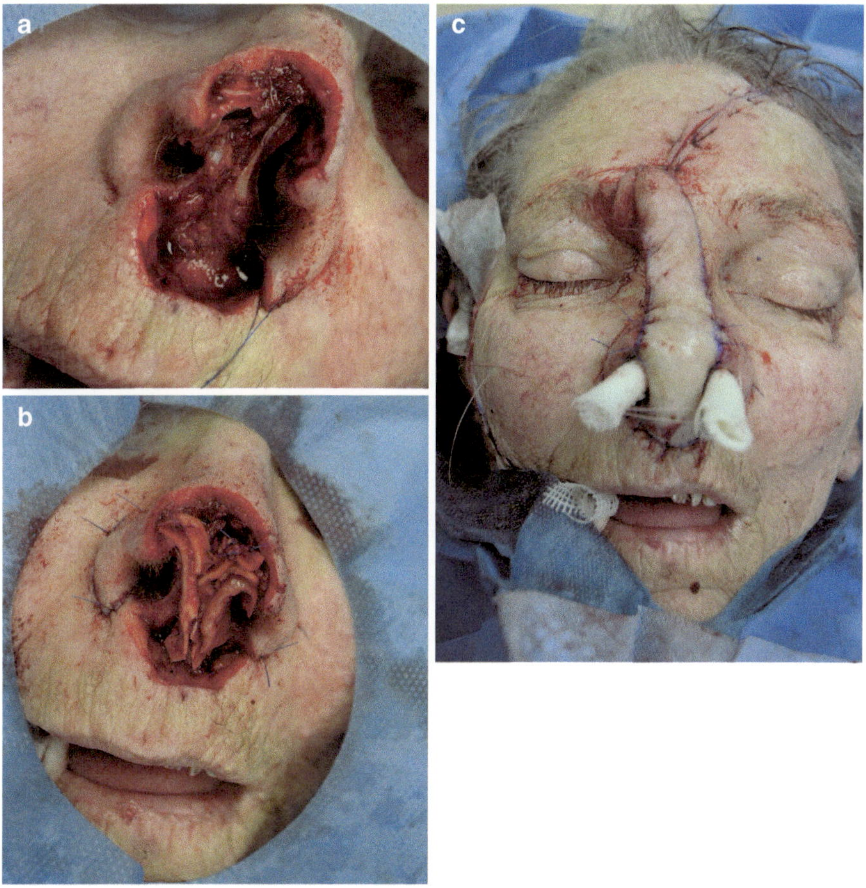

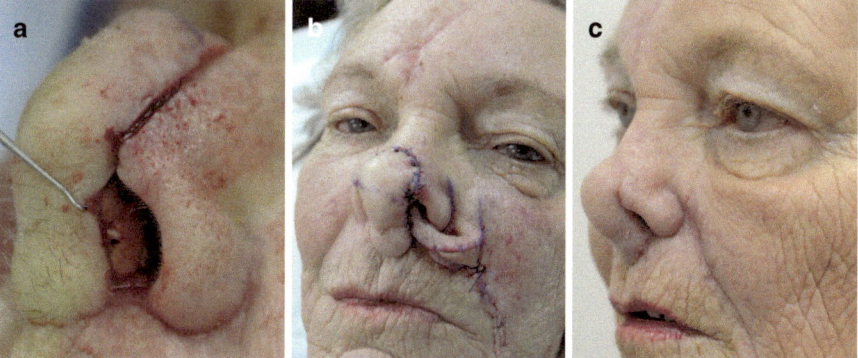

Fig. 18.8 Nasal defect following radical excision of the SCC of the nose (**a**) and stage 1 reconstruction with septal lining mucosal hinge flap, cartilage grafts to construct framework (**b**) and paramedian forehead flap for covering layer (**c**)

Fig. 18.9 Stages 2 (**a**), 3 (**b**) small left nasolabial flap to cover exposed septal cartilage graft and 4 (**c**) to divide and inset the forehead flap and achieve healing of the caudal septum

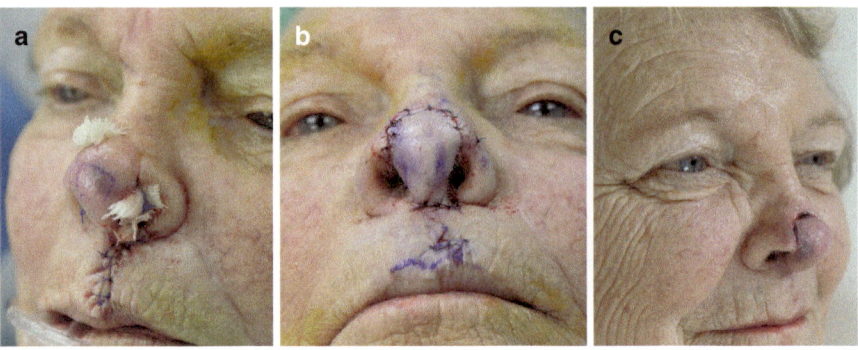

Fig. 18.10 Final stages (**a–c**) to refine and contour the nasal tip with onlay cartilage grafts

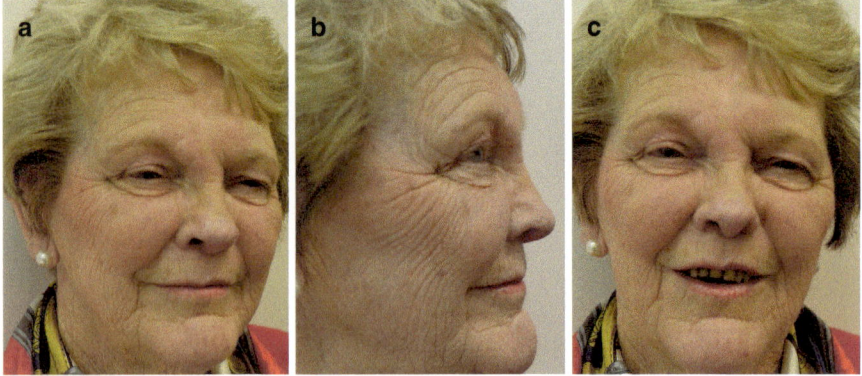

Fig. 18.11 Final result at 3 years and no sign of recurrence

Appendix

Part V

Other Resources Considered for this Book but not Formally Referenced

Australian Cancer Network. Guidelines for the management of cutaneous melanoma. (2008) Sydney: Australian Cancer Network.

Grabb WC, Smith JW (1979) Plastic surgery, 3rd ed. Boston: Little, Brown & Co.

Jackson IT (1985) Local flaps in head and neck reconstruction. St. Louis: CV Mosby Co.

Penington AJ (2007) Local flap reconstruction—a practical approach. Sydney: McGraw–Hill.

Richards AM (2002) Keynotes in plastic surgery. Oxford: Blackwell.

© Springer International Publishing AG 2018
M.F. Klaassen et al., *Simply Local Flaps*,
https://doi.org/10.1007/978-3-319-59400-2

Glossary

BCC	Basal cell carcinoma
FTSG	Full thickness skin graft
KPIF	Keystone perforator island flap
LME	Line of minimum extensibility
LMxE	Line of maximum extensibility
RSTLs	Relaxed skin tension lines
SCC	Squamous cell carcinoma
SMAS	Superficial musculoaponeurotic system
SSG	Split skin graft

© Springer International Publishing AG 2018
M.F. Klaassen et al., *Simply Local Flaps*,
https://doi.org/10.1007/978-3-319-59400-2

Index

A
Advancement flap, 54, 55, 59–62
    bipedicle, 63
    celsus, 45
    dorsal nasal flap, 47–48
    double, 50–52
        H-plasty, 53–54
        V-Y design, 54–55
        V-Y technique, 59–60
    early version, 46
    mucosal, 48–49
    nasalis, 55
    perialar crescentic, 52–53
    sigmoid oblique, 57–59, 137
    single pedicle, 46–47
    upper lip case, 56
    V-Y technique, 61
        closing surgical wounds, 60
        multiple flaps, 62
        releasing scar contractures, 61
Aesthetica, 175–177
    bilateral preauricular skin grafts,
        173–175
    facelift flaps
        extended, 177
        mini preauricular, 175–176
        moderate preauricular, 176
Aspirin, 29
Asymmetrical ellipse, 36
Asymmetrical Z-plasty, 121–122

B
Banner flap, 106
Bilateral preauricular skin grafts, 173–175
Bilateral rotation flaps, 71
Bipedicle advancement flap, 63–64
Bipedicle upper eyelid flap, 83–84
Bipolar diathermy unit, 23
Biwinged excision, 136

Biwinged flap, 51
Bruns-Chirurgischer Atlas, 71
Burow-Bernard technique, 46

C
Celsus advancement flap, 45
Cervicofacial rotation + glabellar transposition
        flaps, 162
Cheek flap, 131
Classical keystone flap, 153
Classical rotation flap, 66
Crescentic ellipse, 36
Cross finger flap, 133
Crown excision, 39

D
Dog-ear excision, 42
Dorsal hand flap, 139
Dorsal nasal flap, 47–48
Dorsal nasoaxial flap, 92, 137
Double advancement flap
    biwinged, 50–52
    H-plasty, 53–54
Double pretibial keystone flaps, 26
Double-Z rhomboid plasty, 125
Drawing tools, 16
Dufourmental flap, 101–102

E
Ectropion deformity, 184–185
Elliptical excision
    asymmetrical, 36
    crescentic, 36
    crown excision, 39
    dog-ears, 42–43
    modifications, 34
    M-plasty, 38

© Springer International Publishing AG 2018
M.F. Klaassen et al., *Simply Local Flaps*,
https://doi.org/10.1007/978-3-319-59400-2

Elliptical excision (*cont.*)
  steps, 33
  wedge excision, 37, 40–42
Extended facelift flap, 177

F
Facelift flaps
  extended, 177
  mini preauricular, 175–177
  moderate preauricular, 176
Fasciocutaneous island flaps, 143
Flint's circle technique, 10–11
  planning, 19
Forehead interpolated flap + cheek rotation
      flap + lip switch flap, 162

G
Glabellar flap, 92, 93, 138

H
Haematoma, 179, 180, 190
Hatchet flap, 107–108
Hinge flaps
  cross finger flap, 133
  nasal lining, 130
  principle, 131
  reconstruction of nasal lining, 129, 130
  cheek turnover flaps, 130
H-plasty, 53–54
Hypertrophic scars, 183–184

I
Interpolated flaps
  bipedicle upper eyelid, 83–84
  with buried pedicle, 80–81
  Charles Nelaton procedure, 77
  paramedian forehead, 78–79
  serendipity, 82–83
  subcutaneous pedicle, 81
  vascular island, 82

J
Jumping man flap, 123

K
Karapandzic flaps, 139
Keystone advancement + chin rotation flaps,
      161–162

Keystone flap, 147, 149–154, 156, 157, 159
  anatomy and physiology, 143–144
  applications
    cheek, 147–148
    foot, 159
    forehead, temple and scalp,
        150–152
    hand, 157–158
    lateral nose, 149
    lower limb, 156–157
    neck, 152–153
    shoulder, 153–154
    trunk, 154–155
    upper lip, 149–150
  from cervical and cheek regions, 163
  design, 145
  surgical technique, 145–146
Keystone perforator island flaps
      (KIPFs), 143
Kite flaps, 59

L
Local flaps, 6
  aesthetic subunit principle, 8
  anatomical landmarks, 11
  aspirin, 29
  case study, 187–192
  classification, 7
  definition, 4
  description, 15
  desinging, avoid tension, 29
  ectropion deformity, 184
  Flint's circle technique, 10
  gentle tissue handling, 25
  haematoma, 179
  hypertrophic scars, 183
  informed consent, 21
  local anaesthesia, 21
  measure, record and photograph, 26
  oncological considerations, 185
  planning, 8
  precise surgical dissection, 26–28
  principles, 3
  radiation necrosis, 181
  risk awareness and consent, 185
  scar, 8–9
  secondary viral infection, 182
  spare skin, 11
  standard surgical instruments, 23
  sterile technique, 22
  suture without tension, 25
  venous ischaemia, 180
Lower eyelid flap, 93

M
Mini preauricular facelift flaps, 175–176
Moderate preauricular facelift flap, 176
M-plasty, 38
Mucosal advancement flap, 48–49

N
Nasal tip, 192
Nasolabial flap, 77, 137
    inferiorly based, 89
    superiorly based, 90–91
Nikon D3100, 18

P
Paramedian forehead flap, 78, 79, 136
Perialar Crescentic Advancement Flaps, 52–53
Postauricular flap
    inferiorly based, 87–88
    superiorly based, 88–89

R
Radiation necrosis, 181–182
Relaxed skin tension lines (RSTLs, 9
Rhomboid flap, 95–96
Rotation flap, 68–71, 73
    classical, 66
    defect, 66
    to scalp, 67, 135
    skin graft
        for buttock defects, 69
        on face, 70
        neurovascular cheek and lip, 71
        to repair flap donor site, 68
        for repairing lower lip, 71
        subtotal forehead flap, 73
        temporal area, 69
Rotation-advancement technique, 41
Rotationplasty, 65

S
Scar revision techniques, 9
Serendipity flap, 82–83
Sigmoid oblique advancement flap, 57, 58, 137
Single pedicle advancement flap, 46–47
Skin graft
    bilateral preauricular, 173
    for buttock defects, 69
    on face, 69–70
    frontal region, 168

modifications, 72
neurovascular cheek and lip, 71–72
nose, 169
to repair flap donor site, 68
for repairing lower lip, 71
scalp, 167
subtotal forehead flap, 73–74
temporal area, 68–69
upper lip, 171
Skin tumour, 6
Sliding advancement flaps, 136
Sliding flap repair, 33–34
Subcutaneous pedicle flaps, 81
Subtotal forehead flap, 73–74
Surgical plan, 17
Swing-slide plasty, 103–106

T
Technique of halving, 42
Tetrahedral Z-plasty, 119
Transposition cheek flap, 138
Transposition flap, 87–90, 102
    banner, 106
    Closure, 87
    critical length, 86
    dorsal nasoaxial, 92
    dufourmental, 101–102
        vs. rhombic, 102
    glabellar, 92
    hatchet flap, 107, 108
    lower eyelid, 93–94
    nasolabial
        inferiorly based, 89–90
        superiorly based, 90
    pivot point, 86
    postauricular
        inferiorly based, 87–88
        superiorly based, 88–89
    rhombic *vs.* dufourmental, 102
    rhomboid, 95–97
    square peg, 98–100
    swing-slide plasty, 103–104
Triangular flaps, 110, 113, 117, 119,
        121, 123, 125, 128
    angle size, 121
    bridle scar, 117–118
    double-Z rhomboid plasty, 125
    jumping man, 123
    notching of lip, 117
    scar revision planning, 116
    W-plasty, 127
        effects, 128
        rhomboid to, 125

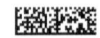

Triangular flaps (*cont.*)
  Z-plasty
    asymmetrical, 121
    clinical applications, 113
    finger web, 120
    functional achievements, 113
    initial steps, 110
    modify, 119
    planning, 117
    repair, 123
    tetrahedral, 119
    transposition, 110
    variables, 110

U
Upper lip case, 56

V
Vascular island flaps, 82
Venous ischaemia, 180–181
V-Y technique, 55
  advancement, 61
  closing surgical wounds, 60

  double, design, 55
  multiple flaps, 62
  releasing scar contractures, 61

W
Warfarin, 29
Wedge excision, 37, 38, 40
W-plasty, 127
  effects, 128
  rhomboid to, 125

Z
Z-plasty
  asymmetrical, 121
  clinical applications, 113
  finger web, 120
  functional achievements, 113
  initial steps, 110
  modify, 119
  planning, 117
  repair, 123
  tetrahedral, 119
  variables, 110